"Inventing the Glidescope (video laryngoscope) revolutio... e life-saving task of placing a breathing tube in the trachea. Dr. Pacey's device has preserved oxygenation for patients and eased the anxiety of countless anesthesia providers and emergency personnel when confronted with critical situations. With this book, he draws on his own experience and that of other breakthrough inventors and lays out the steps involved in getting a medical invention from idea to product."

Michael J Bishop, MD, professor emeritus of anesthesiology and pain medicine at the *University of Washington*

"Although Dr. John Pacey describes the development of a significant medical invention, his book is an important and practical guide for anyone with an inventive mind and an aspiration to build a high tech company. After a long and very successful career as a vascular surgeon, Dr. Pacey made a conscious decision to become an inventor and develop solutions to numerous problems in his field of practice... No matter the field of experience and expertise, this book is a must read for any inventor or entrepreneur looking for a similar road to success."

Michael J. Jervis, B.Sc., retired telecom industry executive and former dean of electronics and electrical engineering at *British Columbia Institute of Technology*

"Medical inventors are rare and rarely deterred—even when working in medicine's conservative environment. Dr. Pacey is one of those—a surgeon determined to provide a better tool for other medical specialists—a preposterous and presumptuous idea, yet revolutionary. This book helps explain why this inventor and others like him needed to push the limits and describes some of the obstacles they overcame. I had the privilege of being at the side of two of these individuals (Pacey and Brain) during some of their discoveries, and it is our good fortune that they are wired differently from the rest of us."

—Richard M. Cooper, B.Sc., M.Sc., MD, FRCPC,
professor on the faculty of medicine at *University of Toronto*

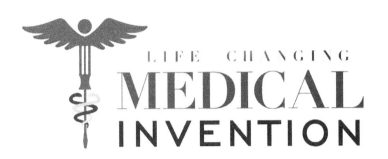

LIFE CHANGING
MEDICAL
INVENTION

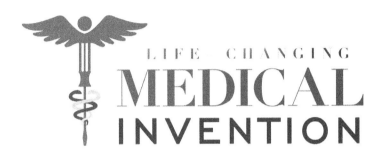

LIFE CHANGING

MEDICAL
INVENTION

Build a **SUCCESSFUL ENTERPRISE** *and a* **NEW WORLD**

DR. JOHN ALLEN PACEY, MD, FRCSC

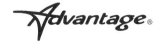

Published by Advantage, Charleston, South Carolina.
Member of Advantage Media Group.

ADVANTAGE is a registered trademark and the Advantage colophon is a trademark of Advantage Media Group, Inc.

Printed in the United States of America.

ISBN: 978-1-59932-666-5
LCCN: 2015942306

This publication is designed to provide accurate and authoritative information in regard to the subject matter covered. It is sold with the understanding that the publisher is not engaged in rendering legal, accounting, or other professional services. If legal advice or other expert assistance is required, the services of a competent professional person should be sought.

 Advantage Media Group is proud to be a part of the Tree Neutral® program. Tree Neutral offsets the number of trees consumed in the production and printing of this book by taking proactive steps such as planting trees in direct proportion to the number of trees used to print books. To learn more about Tree Neutral, please visit **www.treeneutral.com**. To learn more about Advantage's commitment to being a responsible steward of the environment, please visit **www.advantagefamily.com/green**

Advantage Media Group is a publisher of business, self-improvement, and professional development books and online learning. We help entrepreneurs, business leaders, and professionals share their Stories, Passion, and Knowledge to help others Learn & Grow. Do you have a manuscript or book idea that you would like us to consider for publishing? Please visit **advantagefamily.com** or call **1.866.775.1696.**

TABLE OF CONTENTS

INTRODUCTION

THE JOURNEY

This book is the story of a deliberate journey into the world of invention and innovation. The second part of my professional life was a gradual transition from being a busy and successful vascular and general surgeon to becoming CEO and cofounder of a medical start-up, Saturn Biomedical Systems. Awni Ayoubi and I shared the enthusiasm to begin to develop a medical technology company.

Great credit must lie with my small family of origin, starting with my mother who died at age 37 from breast cancer and to whom I pledged that I would become a surgeon. This pledge came from the sense of powerlessness I experienced at age 20 as my mother lay encumbered by advanced metastatic breast cancer. I was angry and needed to give her something meaningful when all she cared about was my future. This pledge changed my life.

My father, Jack Sr., who himself was a restless innovator, created a professional career as an industrial and aerial photographer that greatly improved his life. Watching his determination to achieve was, on reflection, a powerful influence on my own restless approach to life. His notion to always be useful and "add value" was a good one. "I have a thousand ideas" was his favourite saying. From his example, I was always fired with an enthusiasm that I seemed able to project to others during my multiple careers.

The operating room is a special place. The surgeon sets the pace of expectations and creates the work environment. That environment can be a negative one (rants or, times past, throwing tantrums) or a positive one, where the surgeon creates a great environment and the staff enjoys a hard day of work and thanks him for the day.

The path to a surgical career was not an easy one for someone who started education in a rural school that had never produced a university graduate of any kind and where there were 19 students in eight different grades, but I was able to graduate in medicine in 1967 in the upper third of my University of British Columbia (UBC) medical class.

My determination to succeed was tested in the second year of surgical training where, as resident surgeon, I arranged surgery for free clinic patients and started the operations until, at some point, the staff surgeon appeared. Early one morning I began a cholecystectomy, or gallbladder removal, with the help of a student nurse. I made a 30 cm incision from the xiphoid to the umbilicus and was beginning to dissect the gallbladder from the liver when the surgeon—also the head of the resident training program—appeared and immediately began directing me to follow a path that I could not easily understand. I carried on with my plan, which I believed to be absolutely correct. In frustration, the surgeon picked up a scalpel, threw it toward the Mayo stand and the student nurse, and departed from the operating room, apparently furious. The student nurse fainted. Shaken by the outburst, I asked the circulating nurse to call for the chief surgical resident to help me complete the surgery. This we did, and I believed that this event was going to mark the end of my short surgical career. The patient survived the operation and had an uneventful recovery.

The staff surgeon developed a severe headache after he left the operating room. He was encouraged to go to the emergency department for evaluation, where it was discovered that he had secondary brain metastases from lung cancer. He had a long smoking history. Thus was I spared from an ignominious exit from surgical training. Thankfully, I was resilient enough to carry on under fire.

My early career as a surgeon gave some hints of my inventive nature, as exhibited by an incident when I was a member of the Vancouver General Hospital ICU Shock Trauma Team with orthopedic resident Dr. Tony Preto. The shock trauma team concept had been derived from the experience of the Vietnam War, which had demonstrated the value of early helicopter evacuation and rapid infusions of saline-like solutions for patients in shock. The clinical entity of Da Nang lung was an offshoot of this aggressive treatment strategy, because many more patients survived transport only to experience extreme lung "white out" from overinfusion of non-colloid solutions. ICU Shock Trauma focused on aggressive resuscitation, but we were prone to the administration of whole blood or blood fraction products in our civilian hospital. Virtually all Vancouver General Hospital (VGH) severe shock patients had initial therapy by our hands.

While on this team I was called to the emergency department to treat a patient with cyanide poisoning. I knew nothing about cyanide except that it went intracellular and destroyed the cytochrome oxidase system, the final pathway for oxygen use in the mitochondria, resulting in death. I reasoned that there would be no point running to the emergency department with so little knowledge, so I walked toward the emergency department, consulting the Bible of drug treatment, *Goodman and Gilman's Pharmacological Basis of Therapeutics*. The book describes a cyanide poisoning kit, which protects hemoglobin by forming meth-hemoglobin to bind circulating cyanide. On arrival at the emergency department, I put the book down and called for the kit, which to my surprise was available. With an out-of-the-box thought, I called Dr. Bill Trapp, a thoracic surgeon who was the head of the West Coast Hyperbaric Chamber Facility. I reasoned that hyperbaric oxygen might deliver extra oxygen to the cells when the standard hemoglobin delivery system was disabled. The cyanide kit contents were administered and the team rushed the patient through the tunnels of VGH to the hyperbaric chamber. The patient became conscious immediately with two atmospheres of pressure. This proved to be the first recorded use of hyperbaric oxygen for the treatment of cyanide poisoning.

The patient had been robbing a goldsmith when he jumped into a cyanide bath to escape police dogs. The cyanide produced seizures with opisthotonos, or severe rigidity, arching of the back, and hyper-extended distal extremities. The patient made a full recovery and an alert anaesthesia fellow reported the case at the First European Congress on Hyperbaric Medicine in 1983.

My interest in inventive thinking reaches back to 1995 when, on a flight from Boston, I read an editorial in the *Economist* magazine that described the post-2000 future as "dominance of the world of ideas over production." This implied that the largest value would be created when invention and innovation were harnessed to replace older, less efficient technology. Production could be done anywhere in the world. I decided to become a medical inventor.

Thus, I became enthused about intellectual challenges and obtained a new outlet for my curiosity. Invention is based on the Latin word *invenier,* meaning "to find or discover a new device or process that has not previously been conceived." An invention is often the result of an individual working alone or with a small group in an informal venue. A garage is the classic example. An invention, by its unique-ness, has no market and must overcome existing doctrine to appeal to early adopters.

Innovation is derived from the Latin *innovatus,* meaning "to renew or change." This is often confused with invention but is distinct. Innovation is the serial modification of an invention or a number of inventions to create a stream of increasing value.

The Post-it note is an example of these definitions. The original invention by a 3M employee was accidental. In 1968 Dr. Spencer Silver, a 3M scientist, was attempting to develop a super strong glue when he serendipitously developed a weak glue that was reusable with low tack pressure. The glue, while a disappointment, was not abandoned but used by Spencer to tack memos in the lab. While there was little interest within the 3M business development office, lab workers used the product regularly. The ubiquitous Post-it was introduced in 1977 as Press 'n Peel, with a poor response. When it was rebranded as the Post-it note in 1980, success was achieved. This highlights the importance of product names that have resonance and power in the marketplace.

Innovators must know enough about the market needs and the strength of the idea to understand that their solution is the best or one of the best available. The inventor must propel the idea until there is evidence that it is strong enough to build a company and become the "golden offering." Inventors must cast off less worthy ideas and projects or risk spiralling downward into a bankrupt abyss. The enthusiasm of the inventor is needed to build a team to provide skills, money, encouragement, marketing, and positive forces that feed the growing idea. Conversely, supporters will vanish should the inventor-messiah lose firm commitment to the idea. The degree of financial loss experienced will be accentuated if a failed idea is pressed too far. The true inventor is not afraid to move on to another idea or project because it is the intellectual journey that fires the imagination.

The judgment of the inventor clearly will be important here. He or she will see what others don't and will have much more knowledge to judge the validity of the project. The inventor becomes a salesperson to convince others to believe in the idea. Investors want to see that the inventor has attracted quality people to the team because a great team will often find a way to overcome obstacles and produce a successful conclusion. A good team aligned to attack a significant problem will be likely to find a good solution. Should they have difficulty, they will reconfigure to make another attempt, whereas those with less skill will flounder in adversity. Never work with obnoxious, abrasive, untrustworthy people as employees, partners, customers, investors, or consultants. To do that is to risk grinding your business and people in a very negative way.

Investors know that while the inventor has a critical cheerleader role to play, it is only by *forming a powerful team* that success can be achieved. This remains true and gains validity as the growing company increases the tempo and needs more experienced decision making at many levels. The power of talented people may seem to be obvious, but this power is usually not fully appreciated until you have the experience of watching great people working on behalf of your idea.

PHYSICIANS AND INNOVATION

Physicians are a highly selected group of individuals who have intelligence, drive, problem-solving ability, and, at times, inventiveness. The desire to invent may lie just under the surface and, at times, cries out for expression. Similarly, professionals such as dentists, engineers, and other highly educated individuals may hold inventive impulses.

Physician training is like most professional training programs. Educators take a highly motivated young person, hopefully with a generous aliquot of will to "help others," mixed with a determination to make a contribution, and they initiate a mass data dump onto the hungry student. This data dump is coupled with a decision-tree style of training to produce a reliable technical expert who will apply current thinking and knowledge.

Professional training tends to take the curious mind and first assure discipline that will deliver the "known benefits" of a scientific art. The moments of creativity are, typically, extinguished in a drive to create an educated, predictable expert. The creative will is trumped by the collective learning of the medical community. More recently, medical schools have begun to recognize the need for a more open-minded approach, but few medical schools have a real curriculum in innovation. This is a hypothetical example of what one could look like:

What You'll Learn on the UBC Medical School Innovation and Entrepreneurship Track

Following an intro to innovation and entrepreneurship, you'll take three required modules, one track-related elective, and one free elective. Courses include: Prototyping, Qualitative Models, Consumer Behaviour, New Product Development, Disruption, Selling Your Idea, and Social Entrepreneurship.

A new goal for the medical school could be to have the highest number of patents and successful products generated by its graduates.

The emergence of divergent creative thought in medical graduates and students is viewed as a high-risk activity. The usual response to creative thoughts is assurance that the conventional wisdom is likely correct, you are likely wrong, and, for your own good, "don't experiment with your patient." The inventor is therefore regarded with scepticism as well as mistrust.

The new physician should be a very adaptive individual who can venture into the worlds of inventiveness and organizational management in a more effective way than in the past. Physicians are undergoing pressure for change as the health-care system matures. The individual is critical in change management and execution. Individuals make remarkable contributions when trained to anticipate change and embrace it. The physician change manager is a concept whose time has come.

This book is intended to provide building blocks for the medical inventor or medical CEO and will attempt to outline some major topics that need to be understood.

LESSONS LEARNED

- Medical curriculum course content in innovation is urgently needed to enlighten medical graduates about innovation and the business of innovation.

- Determination and passion are essential for success in innovation companies.

- The physician change manager is a concept whose time has come.

PART ONE

INVENTORS AND INNOVATION:
WHY DO THEY DO IT?

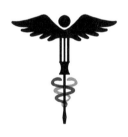

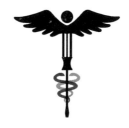

CHAPTER 1

THE PHYSICIAN INVENTOR: DREAMER, MISSIONARY, OR GENIUS?

Who are you, and why are you driven to invent? Understand these questions before you make the plunge to enter the innovation world.

The first task of any person embarking on a complex journey is to answer the question, who am I? There are four recognized possibilities for the entrepreneurial DNA of the individual.

1. Builder, Bulldog DNA is the person driven to grow a company.
2. Optimist, Greyhound DNA is the rainmaker, opportunist, looking for glitter.

3. Specialist, Golden Retriever DNA is the perfectionist person with love of detail.
4. Innovator, Border Collie DNA just wants to create new ideas and be a free thinker.

Find out your natural DNA, and apply that knowledge to the task of finding the matching personalities needed to develop your team. Consult the book *Entrepreneurial DNA* by Joe Abraham.

Medical inventors or engineers becoming CEOs ideally have some qualities required for leadership, but the range of capabilities a CEO needs is daunting. Toughness, determination, and persistence must be matched with a large base of new knowledge.

Ethics should determine how you move forward.

The Hippocratic Oath is an early pledge to first do no harm. Those who develop drugs, devices, or procedures that inevitably have both positive and negative features are necessarily accepted on a balance of good over evil.

Never compromise your commitment as a physician to advance your medical mission. At least two streams of commitment are in conflict as you embark on an inventive career. You must wear the business leader hat at the same time as your medical hat. You could argue that your judgment is compromised by the very existence of this dual role. I would say that you are committed by oath to first do no harm and act in the interest of your patients at all times. Therefore, you must honestly recuse yourself from some decisions in the interest of patients and also investors. Ethically, you may not proceed in this role should you be seriously compromised in the chosen business path.

As an aspiring inventor, you must begin with the notion that you are a work in progress with growth requirements in all categories. The steep learning curve is assured. What attempts have been made in the past to address the issue that you have chosen to try to solve?

The Internet and electronic media have made knowledge widely available and difficult to protect. As an aspiring inventor, your best defense may be your lack of recognition and "under-the-radar" anonymity. The search for a great idea must be carried out with care to avoid donating your intellectual property to the world while, at the same time, getting access to people and knowledge rapidly. Google searches with keywords, YouTube searches of current practice, basic science references, and current practice sites can all rapidly yield information. Preliminary knowledge and a sharp mind can often qualify an idea as previously invented, additive to existing knowledge, or unique with the potential to make a patentable contribution.

Complement your DNA by careful choice of a cofounder. Disclose your idea and inspire the potential collaborator but proceed under nondisclosure coverage to get complementary skills to join what I call the "army of the willing." Presentations in public forums such as a university class or study session are not a good idea. Such groups are unlikely to give useful feedback. Should they do so, you would be exposed to a claim on the idea. Talk with no one unless confidentiality has been pledged and an assessment of character has been undertaken.

It is important to know what you know and don't know. The typical physician is focused on patient care, practice development, practice knowledge enhancement, and solving the problems of the specialty area. This is not what is required of a physician knowledge manager in a new business, who must learn the skills of "idea management." You need not invent this, but study the work of thousands of others who have successfully walked this path.

The physician may be actually impaired by proximity to the orthodox sciences of medicine. There is usually no pain with the status quo. Paradoxically, the great emphasis on proven procedures limits the inquiring mind and makes experimentation more difficult to justify. The entry of government in this equation further complicates the process for the inventor, as government bodies have great weight and little flexibility. The FDA super-regulator has the daunting task of encouraging change while protecting the innocent.

The attractiveness of medicine as a profession has been constant over the ages and, thankfully, attracts those of intelligence, drive, passion, and a desire to live by the Hippocratic Oath, which prescribes "first do no harm." All physicians of experience know that therapies balance good and harm, so decision making demands evidence and clinical experience support. Physicians derive the greatest reward from the direct patient contact they have in their medical practice. The increasing interference of government systems and bureaucracy detract from freedom and satisfaction, causing "burnout" to be common.

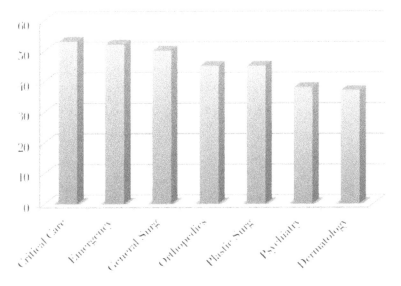

Fig. 1:
The physician burnout percentage may, paradoxically, be a potent cause of inventiveness. Physicians often wish to be left alone to provide for their patients in a direct relationship. Some will react to bureaucracy by getting an MBA and becoming an administrator. Many will react with resignation, while others will look for a creative exit.

LESSONS LEARNED

- Medical teaching encourages young physicians to operate in the channel of conventional wisdom so patients get the benefit of evidence-based medicine. Departure from convention in medical school is treated with a sharp slap that moulds the student toward conformity.

- The need for midlife invigoration can be fulfilled by taking a creative path by use of intellect to create new ideas and devices.

- What got you where you are today will not get you where you want to go. It is imperative to embark on a self-directed learning program for life.

- Choosing to become an inventor is fundamentally different from deciding to pursue a specific goal or mission because the focus is to be free to exercise passionate creativity.

- The physician who becomes a knowledge manager in a new business must reach out to learn the skills of "idea management."

- Know your DNA, and use this knowledge to choose cofounders or collaborators.

- When you begin your business and inventive journey, do not work with mean, obnoxious, abrasive, or untrustworthy people as employees, partners, customers, investors, or consultants. Toxic people will grind you, your business, and your staff.

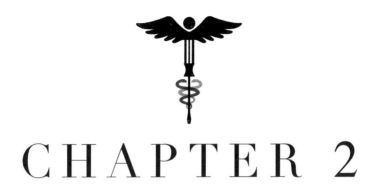

CHAPTER 2

BIOTECH INVENTORS

This discussion of biotech trends is an attempt to understand the nature of the inventive process and of the inventors involved. Serendipity is important, as is the role of a planned and determined analytical path toward invention.

The pace of change and availability of information propelled by the Internet network enables a great many entrepreneurs to enter the health field. The speed of collaboration has been accelerated by network-induced knowledge velocity whereby it is possible to directly contact the most active thinkers online in seconds.

There are many examples of new-age biotech inventions, including some of the work being done by Apple and Google to create health ecosystems. Health ecosystems are gaining complexity at an astounding rate as hundreds of companies toil to provide sensors that measure human function and, increasingly, add predictive software to give us personal health dashboards. I have chosen one of the most remarkable biotech companies as an example to provoke thought.

THE EXAMPLE OF ELIZABETH HOLMES AND THERANOS

Elizabeth Holmes is founder and CEO of Theranos. This company was started to foster application of microfluidics, microanalytics, and advanced technologies in an effort to revolutionize the laboratory testing industry. Laser etching of fine channels allows blood micro samples to be fractionated into fine columns that can be tested with newly created proprietary biochemical testing micro processes. The technology implementation is described in US Patent 8,883,518 B2, "Systems and Methods of Fluidic Sample Processing" of Roy Shaunak, M. Takahashi, I. Gibbons, E. Ku, T. Dang, T. Burd, A. Vollmer, and E. Holmes (Nov.11, 2014). The device designs required to dilute and manage such small blood samples are defined. The array of possible applications is also described in an impressive list. The testing of such small specimens borders on nanomedicine and theranostics. The latter is the combination of nanodiagnostics and nanotherapeutics, envisioning the use of nanoparticles to access the cells and their organelles.

Holmes's work will lead to a massive reduction in cost and marked improvement of availability of medical testing. Theranos technology requires single-drop samples of blood, which are much easier to obtain without patient pain and discomfort and may be taken by relatively unskilled workers or even patients themselves! This trend will eventually extend to the use of sensors that will percutaneously access the fluids of the body and allow their display on computing devices. The Theranos concept has such strong believability that a willing army of investors and supporters enabled ten years of intense work to be carried out "under the radar." It has been called the biggest biotech company you have never heard of.

Holmes's great-great-grandfather was the Danish-born physician Dr. Christian R. Holmes, dean of medicine and surgeon inventor at the Cincinnati College of Medicine. Dr. Holmes created both Cincinnati General Hospital and a psychiatric hospital in Florida. He was a decorated WWI soldier as well. Dr. Holmes's funding efforts were legendary. After reading about his achievements, his great-great-granddaughter decided to commercialize a microfluidic-based laboratory system. Her company, founded in 2003, has a stock value in excess of US $9 billion, based on disruptive innovation in laboratory medicine. Theranos seeks to launch its laboratory system via an agreement with Walgreens, a large retail drugstore chain in the USA that already provides a number of quasi-physician services and point-of-sale services. Holmes was recently asked, why Theranos? She said in response, "I do this because systems like this could revolutionize how health care is delivered. And this is what I want to do. I don't want to make an incremental change in some technology in my life. I want to create a whole new technology and one that is aimed at helping humanity at all levels, regardless of geography or ethnicity or age or gender." This development also threatens the classic physician-based method of delivery of health care.

GENERAL LESSONS

- The Holmes family history inspires the future in a dramatic way with a legacy of achievement.

- The advent of Theranos Medical, led by 19-year-old Stanford dropout Elizabeth Holmes, demonstrates the openness of the inventive landscape. You can dream of developing a BHAG (big hairy audacious goal) and executing it successfully.

- The increased ability to explore and develop new ideas coupled with the networking of people with access to resources can validate an idea and produce a prodigious volume of new and creative technology.

- The Theranos technology is related to the incipient blending of nanodiagnostics with nanotherapeutics in the new field called theranostics.

- Personal health ecosystems are proliferating as entrepreneurs develop sensors to provide input for personal dashboards created by Apple, Google, and other platforms.

- Why is this relevant to the medical inventor? In theory, physicians are forearmed with substantial domain knowledge. The application of this knowledge is limited only by the attitude of the MD.

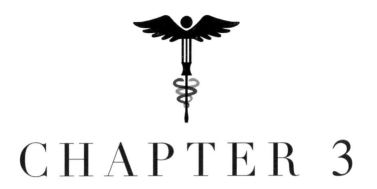

CHAPTER 3

THE INVENTION OF THE GLIDESCOPE

The GlideScope story illustrates the serendipitous nature of invention, the need for tenacity, the value of an effective core team, the value of connecting with key opinion leaders, the value of bootstrapping, and the value of not going forward until there is virtual certainty of the validity of the product concept.

The invention of the GlideScope video laryngoscope will be described here in detail. It will include the thought processes leading to this invention in airway management technology and will explain how a vascular and general surgeon invented a disruptive device in the field of anaesthesia.

The GlideScope video-enabled laryngoscope has led the adoption of video as a means of substantially solving the age-old problems associated with difficult airway management in anaesthesia and critical care. Dr. Alan Klock, professor of anaesthesia at the University of Chicago, reported in the September 2013 newsletter of the American Society of Anaesthesiologists that the development of the GlideScope highly angled video laryngoscope "has led to a paradigm shift in airway management."

LIFE BEFORE GLIDESCOPE: THE DECISION TO BECOME AN INVENTOR

The story begins on a flight from Boston to Vancouver in the mid-1990s when an article in the *Economist* magazine prompted me to thought and action. After 20 years of active surgical work, I was ready for a change. *The Economist* expressed the idea that, after the year 2000, the "world of ideas" would be pre-eminent and production could be carried out anywhere in the world. This theme resonated with me. I grew interested in the possibility of inventing surgical products. I wanted to create those that would ease the practice of surgery through some clever, unique invention. Thus, a spark fell on ready fuel. The rationing of services in the Canadian health-care system was also a factor because the lack of operating time and patient beds occasionally results in periods of relative inactivity for surgeons. A key point here is that I made a conscious decision to become an inventor rather than having a good idea and running with it. By choosing to invent, I was able to come up with a lot of ideas without being wedded to any of them. I was free to drop an idea and exercise my brain on another instead.

I began thinking and before long produced an idea list for product development. My ideas included a harpoon-style anchor stitch for hernia patches, a series of super secure heavy-duty clips for vascular and general surgery blood vessel ligation, a secretion-clearing endotracheal tube, and a series of deployable hernia patches that were designed to permit interventional radiologists to repair inguinal hernia defects with ultrasound or X-ray imaging. I had ideas for ventral incisional hernia repairs that would simplify patch delivery using laparoscopic tools. In addition, I thought of a laparoscopic trocar that would prevent tissues or fluids from obscuring the view obtained by a direct-viewing laparoscope.

LYMPHEDEMA

The vascular surgical problem set includes vexing conditions broadly called lymphedema. I invented a unique new concept for treatment that earned a US patent. This device, made from heavy-strength urethane material ultrasonically welded by local SEI Industries, relied on a hydrostatic column of water on the outside of the leg to counteract the standing column of blood from the heart to the legs, which produced the fluid accumulations in the leg. The external water cuff generated a progressive increase in pressure at lower levels of the leg. While the prototype worked to reduce edema in the leg and also the post-mastectomy arm, it was awkward, hard to use, and did not seem like an invention capable of growing a company.

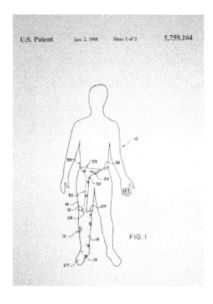

Fig. 2: US Patent 5,759,164 for Pacey apparatus and method for treating edema (Aug. 16, 1995). The hydrostatic cuff concept recognized that leakage of lymph from capillaries was the end result of pathologically high venous pressure produced by a column of blood from the right atrium down to the lower extremities.

This activity led to interest from Johnson & Johnson's Ethicon endoscopic surgery division. A scout came to Vancouver to arrange demonstrations at Ethicon's Cincinnati Research and Development Co-op. This event, circa 1996, was attended by a large group of engineers and project leaders who viewed the application of a trocar-deliverable, radiographic hernia repair device and prosthesis. The devices did not lead to involvement by Ethicon, but a channel was left open for future contact. By this time, I had access to the Jack Bell Research Centre at the University of British Columbia (UBC), which enabled the use of living pig subjects after Ethicon teaching events. This was especially valuable because the lab had instruments, staplers, anaesthesia, and a C-arm for imaging the various interventions. The cost of this work was minimal, because Ethicon provided regular live pig tissue teaching as part of their sales and marketing budgets. Saturn used the tissue only after all Ethicon goals had been achieved. The inconvenience for the Jack Bell veterinary staff was offset with pizza and doughnuts, which apparently more than adequately repaid their work. The veterinary surgery team was also motivated to get as much medical research benefit as possible from each animal sacrificed. I was coached through a certification course offered by UBC to get a diploma in live animal care surgery.

Dr. Alex Nagy, a Vancouver surgeon and head of the surgical team at Jack Bell, was kind enough to enable my years of work at these operating facilities. Later on, when my work crossed into the airway field, the Canadian Army was the unwitting provider of my research animals. The military needed to provide an advanced surgical trauma course for the teams going to the Canadian Expeditionary Force hospitals in Kabul and Kandahar in Afghanistan. The high pace of the war in Afghanistan was producing many casualties requiring surgery. These teams, training at the Jack Bell lab, were treating multiple abdominal and thoracic injuries on adult pigs. The wounds were randomly caused by the instructors and serially repaired by army surgeons using the newly acquired Celox chitosan seashell clotting granules and surgical technique emphasizing the use of multiple applications of surgical stapling devices.

Remarkably, after lung resections, bowel resections, groin-penetrating injuries, and applications of seashell coagulant packs, the animals remained alive and well enough for my work to continue for another hour or more. Using these, I was able to do many experiments getting access to the abdomen, thorax, and hernia anatomy for development of percutaneous hernia systems. I also tested secretion clearing endotracheal tubes that acted like a pump to remove secretions from the trachea.

These early period discussions with two friends, Awni Ayoubi and Fred Kaiser, led to the idea of starting a new biomedical company. Engineer Awni Ayoubi and I were the cofounders. Fred Kaiser, owner of two large, multinational power supply businesses, Alpha Engineering and Argus Engineering, was keen to give support. The new company, Saturn Biomedical Systems, was housed in Fred's Antrim building in the same space as Awni's MTI systems power-supply business. The subsequent concept development was done under the Saturn banner. Support from Argus included 3D design and an engineer who eventually became a full-time Saturn employee.

INNOVATIVE VIDEO TOOLS

The Saturn decision to focus on a video retractor system coincided with acquisition of a large stock of outdated endoscopy equipment from the Burnaby Hospital. This equipment allowed rapid prototyping of tools with a video component and enabled prototypes of surgical retractor systems in my home lab. This basement facility had epoxy, a stock of security CMOS cameras from Supercircuits, LEDs, electronic supplies, ready access, and freedom from any regulatory tracking.

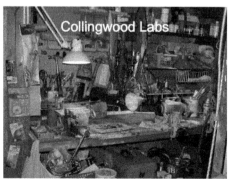

Continuous experimentation produced a large body of notes, reports, and prototypes. It educated the innovator such that when the "serendipitous golden GlideScope idea" did emerge, my experimentally trained mind was able to construct a plan that would prove the concept. Thus, I now emphasize the importance of learning how to be an inventor by working through ideas with tenacity, and yet, with the common sense, discarding ideas not workable in the real world.

Developing ideas becomes a unique journey that develops a new set of skills within the explorer. The toolset will be applied in situations not initially envisaged by the inventor.

The GlideScope's eureka moment was on a day in 1998 when my wife, Doris, and I completed a pig cholecystectomy at the Jack Bell lab using the video-enabled retractor. Later that day, I scheduled a cholecystectomy at Burnaby Hospital. The anaesthesiologists began a 28-minute ordeal using direct laryngoscopy on the thick-necked Italian labourer who had a Cormack/Lehane, grade 4, laryngeal view. The perspiring team used direct laryngoscopy, flexible laryngoscopy, LMA, and Trachlight in attempts to manage this difficult airway. Intubation was finally achieved by blind, direct laryngoscopy. I was scrubbed, masked, and patiently watching this struggle. This loss of control of the airway after the induction of anaesthesia and paralysis of the patient is the definition of a "difficult airway" condition, which is known to be a very dangerous situation and one that has cost many lives and some careers.

Previous work made it obvious to me that the newly invented video retractor could be perfected to visualize the larynx in an anaesthetised patient. I realized that I would need to create a series of video laryngoscope prototypes to get the high performance that would be needed for this challenging task. My surgical experience, which involved the early use of video, made me believe that the introduction of video tools to anaesthesia was inevitable. I was excited about the prospect of getting on with this task.

The GlideScope was then invented at my Collingwood basement lab with an air of great excitement. The first prototype was conceived with a 45-degree arthroscope to look around the tongue and cast light behind it to view the glottis. The proof of concept was carried out on airway manikins. Then a local company machined Delrin and stainless steel prototypes for first clinical use.

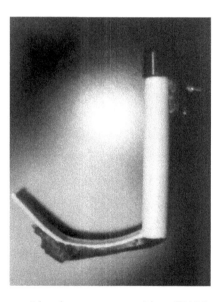

Fig. 3: The first true video laryngoscope with a CMOS camera epoxied at Collingwood Lab.

AN INVESTIGATIVE AGREEMENT THE FAST WAY

The Institutional Review Board (IRB) at UBC approved an investigative agreement for an initial study on patients. This IRB approval established a record by being completed in seven days. I discovered who would need to sign the document and physically searched out the signatories to explain that the project was signed off by Dr. David Bevan, professor of anaesthesia. This aggressive approach was received well by the professors and avoided the usual six-month application process. This IRB due process would never be possible in modern universities where legions of process people govern the rate of change. The new sophisticated procedures attempt to guarantee that all safety measures have been taken and documented.

The Saturn engineering leader, Fouad Halwani, a long-standing friend of Awni Ayoubi, was looking for new challenges. Although based in Montreal, he commuted tirelessly to Burnaby, British Columbia, solving a multitude of problems that led to the many embodiments of the device. Fouad, a generalist with a singular drive to master all kinds of engineering challenges, produced the engineering foundation for all the great GlideScope products made between 1999 and 2006.

Early GlideScope prototype CMOS cameras were security cameras ordered online from Supercircuits in the USA and incorporated into GlideScope shells with red and blue LEDs, using soldering techniques. Soldering was a problem going forward because of the variability of operators. Variable heat of application produces weld inconsistency, which is the enemy of quality. Later, we were able to design flex circuits that were much more reliable and less costly. The choice of LEDs was limited by the absence of white LEDs in the early days of LED development. The combination was selected from available red, green, blue, and yellow LEDs. The red and blue LEDs of the GlideScope were oddly attractive to users who mused on the color selection, so this became a selling point. We pointed out that the red LED provided good viewing of the mucosal surfaces while the blue provided high contrast for the images. The CMOS camera operated in black and white and produced a very useful grey-scale image. This early device was able to penetrate bloody fluids and render a functional image that consolidated our reputation in difficult airway situations—*the rescues were happening*. The pivotal 728-patient study of Cooper et al., published in 2005, was carried out with this early version of GlideScope.

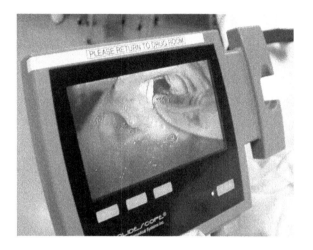

Fig. 4: Early GlideScope airway images.

The need for multiple prototypes became apparent as problems were encountered. If the targets of development are clearly defined as needs of the user and the product specification list is an accurate reflection of this list of user needs, the inventor will go inexorably toward a satisfactory product. All of the inventors described in this book are relentless prototypers. To be an effective prototyper, you need to be a hands-on person because the progressive handwork builds an evolution of knowledge in the brain. This collaboration between the hands and the brain would be akin to the development of skill by an artist, who becomes delighted by effects discovered while working. New ideas flourish during this manual work.

The GlideScope name comes from my flying history as a multi-engine, instrument-rated pilot. When Awni Ayoubi and I were pondering the range of ideas for the name, it appealed to us to call the device after an aviation instrument of the day called the GlideScope. This device gave a picture in the cockpit of the aeroplane's position on the three-degree glide path specified on instrument approach charts. This path takes the aircraft to 200 feet above the runway such that touchdown will occur about 500 feet down the runway.

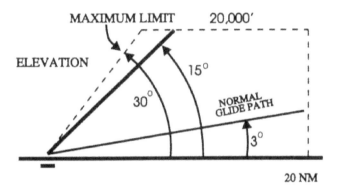

Fig. 5: The three-degree glide path reflected in the cockpit on the aircraft glide slope indicator; the medical GlideScope glides you down to view the glottic opening 99+ percent of the time.

An advisory group was formed, engaging the knowledge of some friends. Michael Jervis had experience as a senior manager in tele-communications and had served as dean of the school of electronic technology at the BC Institute of Technology and was a good friend. Dr. Richard Cooper was professor of anaesthesiology at University of Toronto and an airway expert of renown. Dr. Igor Brodkin was a bright mind from the UBC Faculty of Medicine's Department of Anesthesiology, Pharmacology, & Therapeutics. Fred Kaiser was an established entrepreneur. Importantly, Will Stewart, owner of Vitaid

Ltd., gave Saturn market guidance. All consented to join our advisory board. Igor was assigned by David Bevan to keep track of the project and offer expert advice during development. Support staff was added as the pace picked up. The mission of the GlideScope team was to create a device that would improve the 85 percent success level of the direct laryngoscope to a 99.9 percent success level for the video GlideScope. Thus, a clear objective guided team decisions. Another goal was to make the device effective for cold weather emergency medical service (EMS) ambulance, military, or helicopter applications.

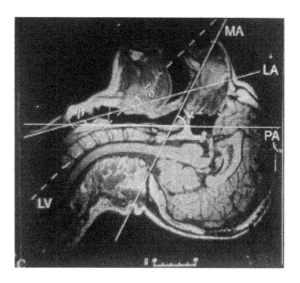

Fig. 6: The GlideScope blade angle of 60 degrees matches the alpha angle created by the intersection of the mouth angle (MA) and the pharyngeal angle (PA). This 60-degree angle permits successful viewing of the glottis 99.9 percent of the time. The failure of direct laryngoscopy is the problem solved by the GlideScope invention.

Seasoned business minds were a critical enabler for the creation of Saturn Biomedical Systems and its subsequent growth. Dr. John Pacey was appointed CEO to fully absorb the liability coming from the patient exploration risks and provide medical decision support.

Then the task of learning to become a CEO was started in earnest, and other chapters of this book describe that journey.

Operational business skills were provided by cofounder and president Awni Ayoubi, whose international experience was of critical importance. Awni's company, MTI Systems, provided many services allowing low-cost bootstrapping to go forward. Argus Technologies, owned by Fred Kaiser, provided Solid Works computer design sub-contracting and personnel seconded for periods of need. Awni's connection to Argus made it easy to access the design assets.

FRUGALITY AND BOOTSTRAPPING

Saturn Biomedical systems success was due to the frugality of the team during the start-up period when the burn rate was contained by the generous supply of sweat equity (work without pay), the relative scarcity of investment money, and the need to avoid large personal financial exposure. The time required to mature an idea and execute a concept is influenced by money availability, but the pace of actual experimentation is what controls the maturation of the product. The longer you can bootstrap on lean resources, the more you can avoid equity dilution.

It is during this early period of start-up company formation that an accurate, timely, and efficient financial accounting structure must be established. It is true that the entrepreneur who carries the burden of financial risk will, of necessity, develop a keen sense of where the money is going by the simple discipline of signing all checks and avoiding credit cards. But an accounting system that produces the full picture when needed and certainly within days of month's end, each and every month, is a primary requirement. When a company has engaged an engineering staff and is making related R&D expenditures, proper and disciplined accounting that has been put in place at the very start of the research process will ensure maximum benefits from the tax authorities. In addition, for planning and budgeting activities, which are so important in the anticipation of cash-flow difficulties (particularly when using the strategy of boot-strapping to reduce the need for capital investment), the budget spreadsheets should replicate the structure of the accounting system. This will provide an opportunity to display the income statement, cash flow, and balance sheet, based on current actual numbers and projected out into future months, based on the specific action plans of the company. It is the capability to see the future in the identical financial format you use when looking at the past that will present the warning necessary to avoid disaster.

Saturn narrowly missed disaster in 2002 when we were burning a modest CAD 30,000 per month early in our marketing and sales drive. The revenue from sales was becoming a significant part of our financial strategy, as sales were brisk. We found that we were able to sell virtually every time we went into the operating room and did our training on real patients. Anaesthesiologists were impressed by the new capability. Because we were light on cash, we decided to raise CAD 200,000 from our personal resources, close friends, and family to give us a cushion. This was timely, because shortly after this round of investment, Health Canada suddenly banned the sale of products from any company not in possession of an ISO 13485 certificate. Saturn was working on this as a low priority, but now we were out of business! The grace period had expired, and we had a lot of work and expense to get our first skeleton of due process in place so that we could pass an audit. We commissioned consultant Karen Delaney to work night and day to make this happen. Had we not increased our cash supply, we would have been desperate and insolvent with an unknown time requirement to pass the audit. This good fortune was luck rather than planning.

The saying, "What got you where you are today will not take you where you want to go," applies here. The surgeon inventor in this case needed to become much more knowledgeable. This required a bottom-up assessment of my personal branding, changing from a surgical helper brand to an inventor hero brand. (Branding will be discussed further in chapter 8.) The hero brand is appropriate for the GlideScope project, because the lifesaving nature of the product often literally produces a heroic intervention. The inventor brand takes its character from this line of thinking.

Mentorship for me came from the advisor group, from the ACETECH CEO group, from President Awni Ayoubi, and later from Gerald McMorrow, CEO of Verathon. McMorrow, a brilliant electrical engineer and Vietnam veteran, had focused on building a superior sales channel for Diagnostic Ultrasound in Bothell, Washington. To achieve this, he maxed out 13 credit cards as a "go for it" financing strategy. The sales channel focus was based on the belief that a good salesperson could be taught the specifics of the product line, but it is much harder to teach sales talent itself. Gerald hired those with demonstrated sales-closing ability and developed what he called his "starving lions" sales force. The power of this sales force was a major draw for Saturn to agree to the Diagnostic Ultrasound purchase. COO Russ Garrison solidly backed up Gerald with extensive medical device operations experience.

The role of Director of Research and Development for Verathon, Canada, was transferred in 2006 to the talented hands of Reza Yazdi, an Iranian-born electrical engineer who proved to be a great credit to his university. Reza came from an anesthesia-focused medical family and had previous experience driving VTech engineering teams in the exacting work of designing low-cost, high-volume telephones. These designs required very low cost of goods, where changes were measured in pennies, and volumes were in millions of units sold. While at Verathon, Reza completed a UBC Sauder Business School MBA with company support, as I believed that he would be a fitting replacement for me at some point.

Reza hired a capable engineering team that was approximately 20 strong. This team was highly productive. The design and development of Canadian-made cameras of high quality and low cost, coupled with the very difficult task of executing the titanium revolution for GlideScope, were some of Reza's highest moments of achievement. Mechanical engineers James Kim and Mitchell Visser made many key contributions during their long tenure with Saturn.

The development of this engineering team was done with great care. Hiring decisions were made after a professional screen by HR consultant Linda Robertson. Excellence in engineering design can only be done by a very high calibre team. It is better to be short of staff than to make a poor hire and deal with corrupted design thinking that will persist in the product throughout its life. Total cost of the product life cycle is baked into the product by the early design choices.

The Canadian company had started to develop product extensions for pediatrics, military, obesity, and disposable products that were designed to avoid infection transmission. This was continued during the Verathon period. Sales grew at a high pace until the product went through US 100 million in annual sales.

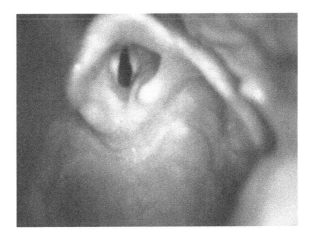

Fig. 7: GlideScope in action giving an excellent airway view.

The Saturn Verathon era resulted in 32 different video laryngoscope designs. Supportive devices were designed such as the Verathon stylets for single and double lumen tubes to exploit video for all airways. Very early, I produced a wireless prototype GlideScope, using Supercircuit cameras, but this was never produced. The Aperture Surgical Retractor project had a halting start, partly because it was in the shadow of the GlideScope, but finally it was also done in a titanium format. This was done over a period of 15 years. These new products incorporated higher-quality cameras made in Canada after a difficult experience with the reliability of digital cameras from China. The Canadian company resisted the suggestions of executives who looked toward outsourcing plastics and electronics from China. We believed we were protecting the Canadian and American economy and workers while producing a high-quality material stream that solved many of the GlideScope's early quality problems. Executives who order apparently lower-cost products from distant sources may be neglecting the cost associated with unannounced component changes that can result in noncompliant product. There are also major problems communicating and connecting with engineering teams that are in different time zones with a different language and different quality priorities. It is far too easy for executives to export our economy to willing foreign hands.

INDUSTRIAL DESIGN: PRODUCING "SEX APPEAL"

My teaching is that 50 percent of device appeal comes from industrial design and 50 percent from engineering excellence. The medical excellence portion of value is a "must have" that is perfected by serial prototyping, verification, and validation.

The importance of industrial design to the success of a product introduction cannot be overemphasized. The value of an attraction to the product, which I have termed sex appeal, creates a willingness to purchase, just for the delight of ownership. This unconscious pride of ownership is akin to believing that you are the best because you belong to a select group that operates at the highest level with the best equipment. Unconscious attraction comes from special lighting, such as blue LED effects, which are reputed to be calming and reassuring. The psychology of a red or orange blinking light is quite the opposite and should be reserved for situations in which special caution is required. Engineers and physicians tend to produce angular objects that speak to efficiency and effectiveness, which may or may not be desirable. Excellence in product and packaging design is proven by Apple to be powerful in the marketplace. To bring in all potential creativity, sometimes it's useful to have an internal/external design contest approach including industrial design experts. Expert industrial designers provide a fresh range of ideas to the executive team. Usually, three choices will be entertained to provide options for consideration.

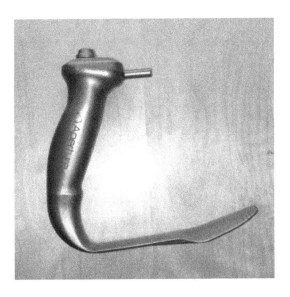

Fig. 8: The titanium Aperture surgical retractor.

One of the most unique and successful Saturn GlideScope designs was the GlideScope Ranger. The military video laryngoscope system was designed after a call from US Air Force Lt. Col. "Boots" Hodge of Fort Detrick, Maryland. Boots had seen the GlideScope at a critical care meeting in the USA. I visited the mobile hospital development center at Fort Detrick, where he requested a compact version of the civilian GlideScope, with the following features. Lt. Col. Hodge wanted a device in the range of 1.5 to 2 pounds, waterproof, able to withstand a six-foot drop onto a concrete runway, functional at 20,000 feet, crush-resistant for light vehicles, and with battery power sufficient to sit on the dock in Kuwait at 40°C for months in a container and then go on a mission without recharge. The mission would involve immersion into salt water, followed by the delivery of power for 30 intubations over a two-week period without recharging.

Following completion of the Ranger, I placed it on the pavement at our Burnaby office to run over it with a Mercedes ML SUV, and then I returned the Ranger to the engineers for successful testing. The Ranger with three hours of lithium battery life went to war in 2005 with Capt. Marvin Friesen of the Canadian Army's medical unit in Kabul. Subsequently, the Ranger served in the prolonged effort in Iraq with US and British forces. The Saturn-designed device ultimately had a distinguished career in Iraq, Afghanistan, the US Marines, US Navy, FBI, US Air Force One, the White House Medical Unit, and US Special Forces. Units have also been sold to the Chinese People's Army's medical service.

The Ranger video laryngoscope earned three honorary battle flags complete with citations of meritorious service:

- The US Army flag (the last medical flag to fly on the last field hospital in Iraq at the date of the US withdrawal).
- The US Marine Corps flag that flew a "dust off" patient extraction mission in Iraq, piloted by Capt. Michael Weathers in a UH-1N Huey USMC helicopter on March 11, 2009.
- The US Air Force flag that flew on a critical-care air transport (CCAT) mission from Kabul to Ramstein Air Force Hospital in Germany.

The presentation of these flags and citations to me from American heroes was very moving and deeply appreciated. The highest honour that I received was from Professor Brian Warriner of the UBC Faculty of Medicine, who recognized the GlideScope contribution by conferring the title of Honorary Professor of Anesthesia at the UBC Faculty of Medicine. I am the only surgeon in that faculty at this time.

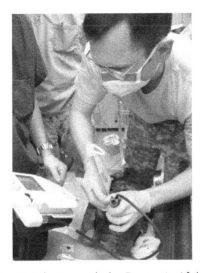

Fig. 9: IED burn patient intubation with the Ranger in Afghanistan.

The penalty for having less than engineering excellence is severe. It impacts the cost of getting the product to the customer and builds up a reservoir of financial pain as product maintenance begins to eat at profits. The more successful the product is in the marketplace, the more costly and more painful this burden will become. This is a lesson that our GlideScope design team needed to learn the hard way.

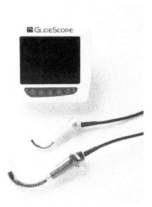

Fig. 10: This image demonstrates single-use adult and paediatric GlideScope versions complete with reusable core camera units and a disposable plastic outer shell of Lexan (paediatric) and K-Resin (adult).

GLIDESCOPE INTELLECTUAL PROPERTY

The intellectual property pertaining to the GlideScope was developed by Ipsolon, an IP firm in Portland, Oregon, recommended by Vancouver inventor James McEwan.

The initial provisional patents were collected into a video laryngoscope patent, Intubation Instrument US 6,142,144 (Nov. 7, 2000), which described a telescopic instrument that embodied a plastic mounting for a 45-degree rod lens endoscope. The patent filed in 1998 was issued after the company had already produced a new-generation, CMOS digital camera product, launched in 2000. The new CMOS work spawned two other US patents, including Intubation Instrument 6,543,447 (April 8, 2003), which captured the notion of a sheath, CMOS camera, LEDs, and an adjustable angle on the lifter arm. The Intubation Instrument 6,655,377 (Dec. 2, 2003) described a heating element for defogging the lens. This patented anti-fog feature was the first use of purposeful heating to prevent fog on the lens of a cold instrument being placed into a hot, moist body. Subsequent patents described a series of sheath designs that were effective in entering the realm of paediatrics and emergency medical service, Video Laryngoscope System and Devices US 2010 261967 A1 (Oct. 14, 2010).

The country selection for the international phase was challenging and limited by budget to approximately six countries chosen by market size and our guess who would try to copy our work. Canada was excluded because the market size is small. Japan, Korea, and China were selected as representative of the large markets of Asia. Brazil and the Eurozone were the other major zones to be included.

The European patents were tested in a Scottish court with a Scottish judge. Verathon alleged that the Scottish company Aircraft Medical violated the Saturn patents. The initial position of Aircraft was that it had developed video at an early date, but our research work investigating these claims clearly proved that the initial work by Aircraft was a redesign of the direct laryngoscope with no video, undertaken several years after the GlideScope had been patented. Although the European Patent Office upheld the Saturn GlideScope patents, infringement was not proven, according to the judge. Because of this decision, the Verathon position was less credible for some notable players who had held back and now were emboldened to compete. Verathon took the position that while increasing the patent portfolio was important, it was vital to treat the competitive process as a horse race in which steady innovation could provide enough value increase to build market share. Verathon's goal to secure the best-in-class status overall was successful.

The lesson here is that an early lead by successful market creation (a truly new product has no market and no competition by definition) must be aggressively followed up by increasing ability to stretch the footprint of the product by forays into new markets. This involves investment in travel and building new relationships with distributors in some areas while establishing full-time sales in others.

Saturn was forced to use distributors in many parts of the world. The advantage of this is lower cost, but the disadvantage is that distributors sell that which is easiest and requires the least investment in time and money on their part. Distributors are difficult to coach on the teaching and training needs of the product, so the message delivered to the customer is variable. The use of distributors to create a change in behaviour and patterns of best medical practice is dependent on the amount of attachment they have to the mission.

The distributor who understands what a disruptive change can do for business development is the one who will invest time and energy. The problem for distributors is that they risk losing the rights to distribute in the future if the product is too successful. The distributor may therefore have mixed feelings about making you too successful, and moderate effort is the result.

The market for video laryngoscopy was created by Saturn Biomedical Systems teaching at major anaesthesia meetings in cities such as Chicago, New York, London, ASA, ESA, and national meetings. Key opinion leader (KOL) work was an important part of our success. We felt that if you are going to get feedback from the key opinion leaders, it's important to get it as early as possible. At a later stage, traditional marketing and "the starving lions" selling team developed by Gerald McMorrow became the most important factors in growth. Multiple doublings of growth occurred as Verathon Medical expanded the sales force in the USA. The market dominance in the USA was based on product performance acceptance along with widespread training at workshops and university training venues. The Seattle US Department of Veterans Affairs (VA) hospital, led by Mike Bishop, and myself from Vancouver, contributed to the landmark paper by Dr. Richard Cooper. In this paper, which appeared in the *Canadian Journal of Anaesthesia* in 2005, Dr. Cooper reported that among 728 patients, GlideScope laryngoscopy consistently yielded a comparable or superior glottic view, and that successful intubation was achieved 96.3 percent of the time, even when it was predicted to be moderately or considerably difficult. Failures to intubate, in this study, usually had an acceptable glottic view. The US VA system became a solid supporter of the GlideScope technology.

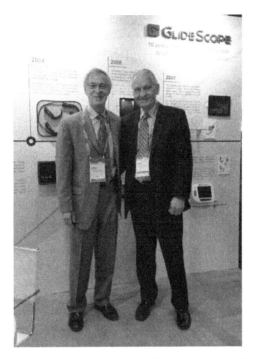

Fig. 11: Professor Richard Cooper with Dr. John Pacey at the World Congress in Buenos Aires, Argentina.

Verathon made a significant investment in the GlideScope for the first few years but later reduced the amount as priorities shifted and investment money was directed at two attempts to establish new brands. The result was a reduction of GlideScope growth. A plastic problem resulted in two FDA-orchestrated recalls. Sales for the reusable devices were stopped in Canada for a time. This was damaging to our reputation and revenue. The new management team, introduced by Roper Industries, decided to press forward with a new and superior titanium product line. It was no less expensive but added sufficient value that the sales leapt forward on a path to maintain market leadership. This demonstrated quite clearly that rather than backing down on price, it is better to add value and quality to serve the customer and the company.

The GlideScope "hero brand" image has been strengthened recently by the determination to build superior quality and long-lasting value into the product. This new thrust will press on in the future in spite of attempts by competitors to enter at lower price points. Maintenance of a brand requires sufficient income to pay cost of goods (COG) with a margin that will allow future research and development, customer service, profit, and penetration into new markets. Customers accustomed to consumer electronics expect complex devices to be available for a few hundred dollars. When they see a specialized device at a higher price, they fail to account for the fact that a typical cell phone is produced in a first run of millions, whereas medical devices are produced in thousands. The regulatory burden is much higher for medical devices.

LEARNING FROM THE SATURN BIOMEDICAL STORY

- The inventor must realize when an invention has great commercial power and take steps to focus on execution.

- Bootstrapping with a small budget is essential to preserve shareholder value.

- Build an initial knowledge base intellectual property (IP) platform with the one-year US provisional patent; the cost is limited to a few hundred dollars. The writing is often done by the inventor. When doing an IP search review of a product, examine how others have solved the problem. Information can be deposited into the provisional US patent document by copying the style of published patents.

- The provisional patent allows marketing of the idea to larger entities, but care must be taken because the effectiveness of the IP at this stage is tenuous, and large entities will not usually help you.

- The IP for GlideScope has functioned for more than ten years as a speed bump for competitors. In the end, however, an innovation horse race strategy was more effective in maintaining the lead. The advantage of being the leader in a field is that the company knowledge base has depth.

- Excellence in reading the customer is critical to the innovation horse race strategy.

- The presence of a strong business and operations capability provided by experienced executives is key to making the start-up viable. The practical implementation requires a person with the company start-up skills of cofounder Awni Ayoubi.

- The GlideScope was successful in powering Saturn Biomedical Systems and then Verathon Medical because it was clinically excellent at solving the unmet need around difficult airway management, and the company had determined medical and business leadership, which joined with key physicians to convince the airway community that this new device was, like the laryngeal mask airway (LMA) before it, a great contribution.

- Do not let perfect get in the way of good to go. When you have verified and validated your specification sheet goals, get the first product into the field where it will provide vital feedback for the company. Prototyping will perfect the product over time.

- Perfection will progressively grow if the company is committed to continuous and progressive upgrading by solving user problems. The current regulatory environment makes this difficult because of the burden of reporting and managing smaller but important changes. This needs to be addressed by the US Food and Drug Administration (FDA) and other regula- tory bodies to allow a more progressive consultative adaptive process. I regard this to be of the utmost importance to get regulators doing what they are meant to do, which is to get the best product in front of the patient.

- The decision to become an inventor is different from the decision to solve a problem. This fundamental difference is demonstrated with Saturn because the inventor motive was to create. The inventor will not be in love with any idea that is unsatisfactory and will tend to abandon it early. This attitude makes the inventor free to move on to something else to satisfy the creative spirit. This could be called innovator DNA.

- The availability of a great simulation, animal, and cadaver lab is extremely important to device developers. UBC has the CESEI facility to fill this role.

- When learning needs become intense, find a great mentor.

- General Colin Powell once said, "Enthusiasm is a force multiplier." This was true inside and outside Saturn and Verathon. A good leader will learn to emit an aura of zeal.

- Financing must be done prior to absolute need. Never run out of money or you will be exploited. Saturn narrowly missed disaster.

- Market dominance must be aggressively capitalized upon to retain the lead. This can be done by progressive product enhancements to sustain product superiority.

- Verathon Medical developed an excellent customer service approach based on the motto of "One call does it all." This was tested later when a series of product-quality issues stressed the services of the company and eroded profitability.

- Weakness in product durability is extremely expensive as the installed base gets larger. At some point this may consume all the energy and excess cash of a growth company. Excellent verification and validation is mandatory. The current Verathon solution is pristine product quality.

- Suppliers as partners in growth.

  ▫ My concept of company relationships with suppliers is to be very close to high-quality suppliers, who then become team members in growth.

  ▫ Supplier insurance methods should be in place. Running out of parts is a huge disaster unless the company can seamlessly shift to gain revenue from another product line. To avoid this, arrange second sourcing in some situations where failure of supply could be due to factors that are permanent, such as supplier business failure. Arranging for insurance by owning excess product inventory defeats the cash return on invested capital (CRI) performance metric by increasing inventory costs. Arrange for inventory to be held by the supplier as a better option.

- Read the financial statement. Sit with your financial advisors to analyze the balance sheet and income statement. Apply the lessons of the CRI indicator. Learn the definition of goodwill and how this will grow to become a substantial part of what you sell when selling the business.

- The cash return on invested dollars or CR is calculated as follows. CRI = net income *plus* depreciation and amortization *less* capital expenditure maintenance. Net working capital *plus* gross property, plant, and equipment (PP&E). This keeps management focused on earning with minimum investment dollars. The CRI goal of Roper Industries is a proven performance driver, because the focus is on steady reduction of investment in working capital, property, plant, and equipment, and inventory while increasing free cash flow.

- The sale of Saturn to Diagnostic Ultrasound was conducted in a suboptimal way that did not maximize Saturn shareholder value. An executive health-related factor and a management team new to this process failed to generate a strategy for the sale.

- View every problem as an opportunity. You will startle your team if you are excited by attacking problems with a super positive approach. Verathon Medical reacted this way when we developed a problem with cleaning reusable Lexan GlideScopes. The problem resulted in a crash program to develop the best laryngoscope in the world out of titanium, the finest metal material in the world. The result was a marked increase in product quality and sales.

- Hire only the best available employees and provide competitive compensation. The price of a poor hire at the executive level can be company failure. Develop world-class human resources (HR) capability and use psychometric testing services to remove some of the subjectivity of assessment. Always interview the ex-boss of your candidate and test the résumé severely.

- Developing a balanced effective approach to Quality Management processes that does not create a burden on profitability is a huge challenge.

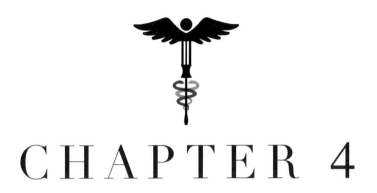

CHAPTER 4

EXCELLENT MEDICAL INVENTORS

DR. ARCHIE BRAIN: PROTOTYPING TO EXCELLENCE–DEVELOPMENT OF THE LARYNGEAL MASK AIRWAY AND THE SGA CATEGORY

Archie Brain was born on July 2, 1942, in Kobe, Japan, the son of the British consul. The Japanese interned the family in December 1941 at the outbreak of the war in the Pacific, and the family was extracted from Japan on July 30, 1942, by a Red Cross ship bound for Lourenco Marques, Mozambique, in a prisoner exchange.

Brain's father wanted him to become a foreign service diplomat, but after completing an honours degree in modern languages at Oxford University, Archie decided to apply to Oxford for medical training. He subsequently went to St. Bartholomew's Hospital, graduating in 1970. This was followed by anaesthesia training at the Royal East Sussex Hospital until 1973, when he was offered a post as chief of anaesthesia at a hospital in the Netherlands. There is a hint here that Archie was impressive as a new graduate and encouraged trust. This led to a British Overseas Development Agency two-year appointment in the Seychelles Islands. In 1980 he returned to London and became a lecturer at Royal London Hospital, which allowed him time to be inventive. In one short year, he produced patent applications for twelve devices. Dr. Brain's great contribution, the LMA patent submitted in 1982, became the foundation for 20 years of effort and prototyping. Without business skills, he failed to find a suitable backer to commercialize the invention. In 1983 he met Robert Gaines-Cooper, who agreed to back the project. Archie was a prodigious prototyper, as are all the inventors presented in this book. He remarked in 2005, at a Society of Airway Management meeting, that the LMA was a 20-plus-year project for him.

Dr. Brain talks about the need for developing communication skills early in the innovation process. Medical innovators need to become excellent communicators because they need to sell their value idea over and over to many people who, initially, may think that the idea is odd. First, innovators need to convince friends and family investors who know them personally but are now being told that their friend or relative is an outstanding inventor who will change the world. Each echelon of new investors is more sceptical than the last. Should an innovator have the good fortune of backing from key opinion leaders, the chances of acceptance improve, but excellence in delivering the sales pitch is critical. Physicians don't usually sell ideas; they explain the clinical situation and allow patients to choose their own fate. The inventor must have acceptance of the invention value proposition or the project will fail. Communication issues lead to failure of a great many useful products and partially explain the 1 percent success rate of innovative ideas in the marketplace.

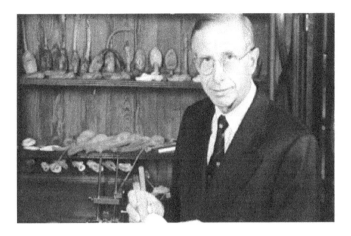

Fig. 12: Archie Brain has a strong sense of history and has preserved an LMA historical prototypes collection. These museum prototypes are a result of early efforts to perfect the laryngeal mask so that it could be safely deployed around the world. The goal was to achieve an excellent record of airway access in easy short cases, then more extended anaesthetics, and finally, difficult airway scenarios. The timing was good because failed airways were not uncommon, and a reliable plan B was desperately needed by airway managers.

The quality of persistence is well demonstrated in the LMA story. The British airway products company Portex initially embraced Dr. Brain. After a year of waiting, it was clear that Portex did not have the same sense of urgency to get the LMA to market. Robert Gaines-Cooper, a Seychelles-based investor who made his fortune in the 1960s by renting and trading in jukeboxes, saw an opportunity. He created the LMA Company with Dr. Brain, which illustrates the utility of joining with a businessperson

The latex rubber LMA was first used clinically in 1981 following development in cadaver models to effectively seal the entrance to the airway. The first publication in the *British Journal of Anaesthesia* in

1983 introduced the device to the greater anaesthesia community, followed by a report of successful use in three difficult airway patients, published in *Anaesthesia* in 1985.

This demonstration in difficult airway work was of great importance to the anaesthesia community. There was a great need for some means of dealing with the "cannot ventilate/cannot intubate" situation that presents the greatest risk to sleeping, paralyzed patients. In 2003 the American Society of Anesthesiologists recognized this capability by including LMA in the revised difficult airway algorithm. This was the first major improvement to the algorithm in its history.

The subsequent development produced a sequence of devices to follow the classic reusables. The devices included Fastrach intubating LMA (1997), Proseal LMA 2000, and the LMA Supreme single-use device featuring an esophageal access channel and easy insertion. The LMA Supreme has a gastric decompression channel, which has earned it a place as one of the most reliable supraglottic airway devices (SGAs) available.

The following paragraphs are contributed by Dr. Archie Brain.

What Have I Learned from the Journey?
by Dr. Archie Brain

Enough to fill a book—which I have yet to write! But as a completely noncommercial person, my greatest difficulty was adjusting my thinking to enable me to understand the commercial world sufficiently to recognize that I needed people with that kind of brain, just as much as they needed my kind of brain to produce the inventions for them. Alone, I would not have succeeded. I also learned that success distorts the way others see you and the way you see yourself. Therefore, I have tended to shun the limelight as much as possible.

My life has been neatly divided into two halves: before the invention and after the invention. My gifts, as perceived by others, had always been artistic, linguistic, and musical. At school I was the typical dreamy poet, hopelessly absent-minded, a voracious reader from the age of eight, winner of solitary activities such as long-distance running or poetry competitions.

When I eventually won a scholarship to Oxford to read modern languages in 1960, an idealistic streak in me came out and I expressed the wish to change over to medicine instead. It was pointed out to me, gently, that I had no obvious scientific abilities and therefore this would be a most unwise step. However, I persisted and was granted a place at St. Bartholomew's Hospital in London, with the proviso that I had to complete my modern languages degree at Oxford first. This I did but with a heavy heart. I felt I was losing time. I struggled to obtain a modest degree, disappointing both my brilliant father and my college tutor, who had been expecting me to get a first-class degree. Then I had to spend time and money struggling to pass the necessary preliminary examinations in basic sciences in Oxford to enable me to qualify to start my medical studies. I hired private tutors and finally, obtained the required grades after an intensive year, working alone. The years that followed were tough too, but I felt I was on the way, without really knowing what that way was to be. In London I started failing the examinations and became chronically sick, finally getting a rather modest medical degree in 1970. I was absolutely thrilled. Then things started to change. Up to that point, it had been not so much black days as black years. Everyone predicted disaster; no one encouraged me. But when I actually became a doctor, I discovered, to my delight, that I really could be effective in this role. There followed some exciting and fulfilling years, but increasingly, I became nervous and unsure where I was heading. In 1973, personal circumstances forced me overseas, first to Holland and then to the Seychelles. I enjoyed the challenges these situations offered, but still there seemed to be something missing. It was not until I accepted a lecturer post at the Royal London Hospital in 1981 that I finally understood that my real destiny was that of an inventor.

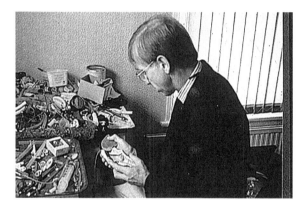

Fig. 13: Dr. Brain working in the mortuary office, building LMA prototypes.

The excitement of inventing the LMA was unbelievable. I was, by now, a very seasoned anaesthesiologist and knew instantly that, as my laconic Scottish professor said to me, "That's a winner." A period of intensive activity followed, yet I was still working alone. Indeed, I continued making and assessing prototypes for the next seven years, gradually discovering what the limits and potentials of this new method of airway maintenance might be, carefully recording all my cases like so many steps in what sometimes seemed like a never-ending staircase.

Were there any black days at all? Looking back, I think the glow of the discovery never really ever left me, so that when I failed to interest the commercial world, this was frustrating rather than depressing. From then on, the main problem became one of communication. I came to realize I had to teach and persuade whole classes of people who knew little or nothing about anaesthesia and what the invention was all about. This included technical information for manufacturers in the USA, France, UK, Singapore, and Malaysia; officials in the newly formed devices department of the FDA; and eventually, distributors in 84 different countries—to say nothing of preparing and delivering lectures in eight different languages.

I have mentioned my professor, Jimmy Payne, who had the good sense to free me from other tasks right from the start. His colleague Dr. John Bushman had a somewhat similar brain to my own, and I owe it to him and to good fortune that when I applied for the job of lecturer at the London Hospital, the professor was absent and it was John who interviewed me. Later on, the number of those who came to recognize the potential of the device increased exponentially, and more and more people started to encourage me, the earliest being Professor Rosen from Cardiff, who gave me my first award, the Pask Certificate. When I was no longer able to continue my job as a consultant anaesthesiologist, I received an honorary appointment at Northwick Park Hospital in Harrow, North London, from the famous British anaesthesiologist Dr. John Nunn, who was pivotal in three ways:

1. He it was who persuaded Mr. Gaines-Cooper that he should do everything possible to commercialize the invention.
2. He undertook the first independent clinical study of the LMA, using my own silicone homemade prototypes.
3. He wrote, introducing me to a number of influential North American colleagues, whom I then went to the

USA to meet, thereby planting the seed of the idea in the Americas.

Finally, I accepted two other important honorary consultant posts:

1. At the invitation of Dr. Chandy Verghese, I came to Reading General Hospital in 1991 where, in a small laboratory next to the hospital (previously an undertaker's premises), I designed and built the Flexible LMA, the Intubating LMA and the LMA Proseal. The testing for all was carried out in collaboration with Dr. Verghese, whose skill and boundless enthusiasm as a teacher of LMA techniques eventually made his hospital a magnet for visitors from all over the world.

2. At the invitation of the director of the National Otolaryngology Hospital in Grey's Inn Road, London, and the chairman of the anaesthesiology department, Dr. Paul Bailey, I accepted an honorary fellowship to study the many uses of the new flexible LMA that had been adopted there as enthusiastically by the surgeons as by the anaesthesia team. Subsequently, this hospital went on to train generations of new anaesthesiologists in the specialized techniques that permit its safe use in the majority of surgical otolaryngology procedures, notably routine tonsillectomy. Sadly, these techniques remain largely unknown outside the UK.

LESSONS LEARNED FROM DR. BRAIN

- Dr. Brain decided to become an inventor and be creative early in his career, giving him time to make multiple contributions.

- Inventors need to be hands-on people!

- Great invention is a life-changing event.

- There always seem to be key mentors or coaches who help get the inventor through dark days when the world does not appreciate the invention. Inventive individuals are driven by a different drummer, a passion to use intellect to create. The inventive mission begins to control the psyche, producing a determination to complete the mission with an abundance of infectious enthusiasm.

- Rejection must be repeatedly overcome by convincing, educating, and selling.

- The opportune meeting with Robert Gaines-Cooper in the Seychelles Islands was later converted into a successful business partnership.

- Companies that try to proceed without high-quality, in-house, medical inventor talent miss many opportunities for modification of products and generating value. Short-sighted executives will fail to understand this because, usually, they are taking to market fully baked products early in their career. They don't have experience dealing with inventive medical input. The nature of medical or any other inventive process requires that many ideas do not work as hoped so they must be massaged into a form that will delight the user or be abandoned.

- The inventor must achieve very high performance from the invention to get endorsement from professional mavens. The LMA was operating in the range of 90+ percent success when introduced.

- Brain created a new category now known as supraglottic airway devices (SGAs).

- Pain points solved by using the LMA routinely included making a hands-on, mask anesthetic procedure into hands-free, reliable ventilation.

- Provision of a solution for the much-feared "cannot ventilate/cannot intubate" situation was a profound change.

DR. MUHAMMAD NASIR AND DR. LUIS GAITINI: LEARNING TO OPERATE IN THE RED OCEAN COMMODITY SPACE

Following the success of Archie Brain, the field of SGA development became very active, with multiple new designs and entrants. Dr. Brain had, however, provided a very durable and effective solution, so the new entrants had variable degrees of difficulty. This situation had become a red ocean or commodity marketplace for inventors trying to get some share of the large market that LMA had created. Seventeen years of patent protection had done its job. In essence, aspirants needed to produce something clearly differentiated to provide a solution to LMA issues. Dr. Brain made this difficult by continued innovation to perfect the device for children, for single-use disposable needs, for EMS use, and for provision of a conduit to intubation as well.

At times, large companies with excellent resources promoted copycat devices, but most of these devices were weak challengers. The world really didn't need them, so they continued to swim in the red ocean. In excess of 15 projects, or roughly one per year, have now been introduced.

Two projects, however, were designed to produce distinctive changes that made a significant contribution. One of these projects has not yet succeeded, but the other has become popular.

THE ELISHA AIRWAY

The first of these was an SGA invented by Luis Gaitini, MD, which I describe as a fourth-generation SGA. This device was constructed through primary reference to CT images, whereas Dr. Brain had used cadaver specimens to get the correct geometry. The Elisha airway device had the following features:

- Like the LMA, it provided excellent ventilation, as shown in a study that appeared in *Anesthesia and Analgesia* in 1999. The Elisha airway device has a gastric decompression channel, like more advanced LMAs, that permits gastric tube placement.
- Like the LMA, the Elisha airway device, in almost all cases, allows intubation via a channel.

- The Elisha airway device had the added advantage at the time of invention that ventilation could be continued while passing an endotracheal tube. This advantage, in theory, makes the device extremely safe in transition from an SGA to endotracheal ventilation.

That the device was in the red ocean area contributed to making it difficult to find a company willing to risk funding commercialization. When the inventor and his primary financing group exhausted their resources, a possible new SGA contribution stalled. The mortality of good ideas is very high, in general, with estimates of failure being from 90 to 99 percent. In the red ocean, this failure rate will climb unless the innovation creates new circles of customers and provides a clear benefit to draw them out.

Dr. Gaitini continues to seek attention for his excellent project, but as time passes, competing devices continue to build market share, so the odds of success are not improving. Hopefully, this will be resolved. A project can be prevented from progressing in so many ways that the most important negative factor can be difficult to define. The people involved are, generally, the most important factor. A high-energy team can have multiple successes and turn around ailing projects. Assembling such a team isn't that easy when resources are limited so the red ocean builds a bias against success.

LESSONS LEARNED FROM THE ELISHA AIRWAY PROJECT

- Finding a compelling added value when in the commodity space is challenging. The Elisha inventiveness created a unique added benefit over the LMA devices. When this was done, a myriad of other obstacles developed, requiring great commitment on the part of the inventor.

- The Elisha airway device was proven to provide excellent ventilation, like the LMA, in a study with multiple authors, published in *Anesthesia & Analgesia* in 2004.

- Investors question projects that challenge mainstream market leaders.

- Never run out of money. Action on the fundraising front must be well in advance of need. Failure of traditional external finance sources means that you must bet it all by sale of assets, increasing debt, and ultimately, risk losing your financial stability. Gerald McMorrow exhausted credit card debt; Dr. Mohammad Nasir sold his house and lived to tell the tale.

THE I-GEL PROJECT

The inventor of the I-Gel SGA also dared to enter the red ocean and challenge the supremacy of the LMA franchise. Dr. Muhammad Nasir noted that, at times, patients suffered from the pressure exerted by the inflatable cuff of the LMA. Many cases of this type were due to absorption of nitrous oxide from the ventilation mixture; others were thought to be due to awkward placement or overinflation. Recommendations centered around monitoring cuff pressure, but this sensible measure was often neglected during the course of anaesthesia.

The approach selected by Dr. Nasir was unique. He reasoned that the mask shape could fit the airway without inflation and thus avoid some injury from extra pressure. He also thought the material used was critical. He decided he needed to find a soft material that had the exact consistency and durometer of the tongue so that the material would be just as likely to deform as the native tissue. The search was not easy. He rejected his first thought, silicone, in favor of a thermoplastic called styrene ethylene butadiene styrene (SEBS), which was a medical-grade plastic with the correct deformability.

Dr. Nasir had an additional problem. The administration of his hospital in his native Pakistan was very unsupportive. The professor told him that he should pay attention to his work. Dr. Nasir found himself in an atmosphere toxic to innovation and creativity. Some years later, while working in England, he was able to find time to refocus on his passion. He spent seven more years on development. He began bootstrapping with self-financing, which ran low very quickly, and heavy use of sweat equity. Using multiple mortgages and selling his house got him to the point where he retained control of the new IP and was able to negotiate a favorable deal with Intersurgical to begin marketing in 2010. The market was very receptive to the new technology.

LESSONS LEARNED FROM THE I-GEL PROJECT

- Dr. Nasir's passion pressed forward with bootstrapping, sweat equity, and extensive prototyping. Success came when he financially leveraged his home to provide capital.

- The least expensive form of capital available to the inventor is sweat equity.

- Single-mindedness over many years is likely to lead to success if all else is aligned.

- Senior people often try to discourage the inventor, so they must be heard but not allowed to stop a great idea with a clear mission.

- The material selection proved to be a make-or-break decision for the project. Good function will allow an idea to generate company-building revenue.

- The willingness to risk it all by mortgaging and selling his house was pivotal in preserving equity, which enabled him to negotiate an excellent arrangement with a commercial partner. This high-risk strategy produces the best financial outcome, but should you make a misstep, you will be starting all over again, with risk to personal relationships and reputation.

- Recent success in the veterinary market has been notable.

DR. THOMAS FOGARTY: INVENTOR, EDUCATOR, AND THOUGHT LEADER

Thomas Fogarty's early contribution to vascular surgery resulted in a dramatic change in management of one of vascular surgery's most vexing problems: embolization and thrombosis of peripheral arteries. Dr. Fogarty's history could easily be the topic of several books dwelling on his experience in conceptualizing new products, mentoring, teaching, and building effective companies.

Thomas Fogarty was of Irish origin. His initial career goal was to be a professional boxer until, in his last year of high school, he suffered a broken nose in a tie match. Tom started from a poor family whose sole earner was his mother. Tom did whatever was necessary to help himself and his family survive. He earned a poor reputation at his school and was only able to enter university because of intervention of a visionary Jesuit priest and his sister, who was dating the vice chairman of admissions. He parlayed this into a successful trial admission to the institution. He decided that a medical career was much more attractive than boxing. He was reputed to be a non-stellar student in the early years, but he was inventive. His early invention and assembly of a centrifugal force clutch for a friend's Cushman motor scooter was a clue of what was to come later. His friend's Cushman was performing badly, so Tom worked with local machinists who, apparently, developed an interest in helping the "kid." Tom demonstrated this fully functional centrifugal clutch to Cushman, and it was adopted by the company going forward without any payment or thanks. Undoubtedly, this experience reinforced his belief in the value of intellectual property.

Dr. Fogarty had a persistent surgeon mentor, Dr. Jack Cranley, who saw his energy and inventiveness at an early stage and provided early encouragement and advice. Cranley brought young Fogarty into the operating room and trained him as a surgical technical assistant, which allowed him to make some badly needed cash. This gave him an opportunity to think in depth about problems he witnessed Cranley dealing with. The inefficiency of the traditional embolectomy surgery first became apparent to Fogarty at this time. He began thinking of alternatives to the traditional surgery, which usually led to amputation and/or death.

Dr. Fogarty began his medical career as an intern at the University of Oregon and completed his surgical residency there in 1965.

At the beginning of his surgical residency, he carried out the first embolectomy on a real patient in 1961, only six weeks after conceiving the idea. The timing here is remarkable. The work was done using techniques he learned as a boy tying flies for trout fishing and by using readily available materials from the urology service in the form of stiff ureteral catheters and latex rubber from the small finger of a surgical glove. To go from idea to first use on patients in six weeks in a complex specialty such as vascular surgery is an achievement that could never be reproduced in the current regulatory environment. The new regulations require a prodigious effort to comply with good manufacturing practices, extensive safety results, and efficacy data. The former era protected the patient by relying on professionalism and concern for the patient. The current world enables an explosive increase in the number of innovation projects, which have a much higher hurdle to be market ready. The regulatory apparatus has grown to control a variety of possible patient risks. These changes slow down innovation but are necessary to prevent patient injury or the existence of poor-quality products in the medical field. To be successful, new products must also qualify for "reimbursement" from insurers or government. The combined effect of these two items is estimated by Fogarty to add as much as seven years to the time required for product development. The US FDA has consulted with Dr. Fogarty to try to streamline this challenging timeline.

LIFE AFTER THE ARTERIAL EMBOLECTOMY BALLOON CATHETER

In Oregon, Dr. Fogarty became acquainted with Charlie Dotter, a professor of radiology who was developing a new technology called interventional radiology. This art is taking the radiologist from being an image reader into a vast new area using the new tools of radiology—angiography, CT, CT angiography, MRI, and ultrasound—to develop a host of new methods of intervention. Examples include draining abscesses, placement of vena cava filters to prevent pulmonary embolism, stent placement, and many others. The concept of gaining access to arteries to carry out dilating angioplasty avoids the extensive cutting and sewing involved in classical surgical approaches. In the beginning, there was strong opposition. Surgeons were very happy with their approaches and regarded the new, minimally invasive strategy as risky and ineffective. The idea was embraced early in Europe but was not accepted in the USA until 1980. Patients often agreed to have the procedures despite negative advice from established US physicians. Dr. Dotter was said to lack tact and was a flagrant showman, somewhat messianic in his approach. He was featured in *Life* magazine with a picture showing glazed eyes. The article scared many and excited some.

Dr. Dotter was considered by some to be heretical and was called Crazy Charlie, but his interest shared with Tom Fogarty was vital for both to speed their progress and development.

Dr. Tom Fogarty began his surgical career at the University of San Francisco as a fellow under the famous Dr. John E. Dunphy. He continued work with vascular catheter systems designed for use in endovascular work.

People who innovate must overcome the orthodoxy around them, and Dr. Dotter was no different. Dr. Dotter requested that Dr. Fogarty be permitted to work with him for a year. The request was flatly refused by Dr. Dunphy, who was a more orthodox surgeon. Dr. Fogarty, however, made the catheters used by Dr. Dotter to perform the first percutaneous angioplasty of a tight stenosis of a superficial femoral artery in an 82-year-old woman in 1964. The two became friends and collaborators. This work led to the first percutaneous transluminal angioplasty (PCTA) of a coronary artery by Dr. Andreas Gruentzig on September 16, 1977.

Dr. Fogarty had a very early start. He developed the embolectomy catheter through a series of prototypes and successful clinical applications. The pace of innovation was high and, soon, the San Francisco hub became a center for innovation success in a way that heralded the Silicon Valley phenomenon to come some years later. The Fogarty clamp was designed for control of large vessels such as the aorta and is now a core piece of equipment for surgeons.

The AneuRx aortic stent graft was invented and perfected by Dr. Fogarty in the early 1990s when he collaborated to introduce the interventional radiology-based approach to treatment of aortic aneurysms.

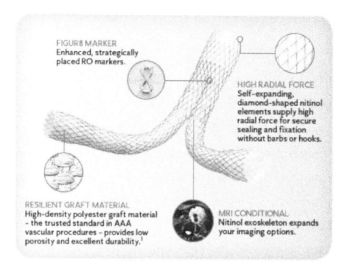

FIGUR8 MARKER
Enhanced, strategically
placed RO markers.

HIGH RADIAL FORCE
Self-expanding,
diamond-shaped nitinol
elements supply high
radial force for secure
sealing and fixation
without barbs or hooks.

RESILIENT GRAFT MATERIAL
High-density polyester graft material
- the trusted standard in AAA
vascular procedures - provides low
porosity and excellent durability.[1]

MRI CONDITIONAL
Nitinol exoskeleton expands
your imaging options.

AneuRx is one of Dr. Fogarty's later achievements. Since its introduction in 1995, there has been an explosion of systems using this principle—and therefore a revolution in treatment of deadly aortic aneurysm disease. Nowhere has this been more significant than in the treatment of a ruptured aortic aneurysm. Traditional surgical treatment is difficult and has a mortality rate in the region of 50 percent. The application of covered stent grafts for aortic aneurysm is now commonplace. While the graft itself is expensive, the savings in lives and hospital critical care resources is overwhelmingly in favour of the technology. The Stanford-affiliated Fogarty Institute for Innovation (fogartyinstitute.org) teaches innovation strategies and allows an incubator-style engagement for small companies. It serves as an education centre for those who need a quick start. Companies that fail to engage excellent medical input are rejected by the Fogarty team as candidates for in-house incubation.

Dr. Fogarty has had challenges with his academic home, Stanford. The occasional medical leadership changes cause new issues to emerge.

He claims to have been fired, or to have quit, Stanford three times over disputes in which attitudes limited his inventive expression.

Within the Fogarty Institute, the Taft Center for Clinical Research aids clinical trials and has an affiliation with the El Camino Community Hospital. Clinical research underway in 2015 is the Trans Catheter Aortic Valve (CoreValve) trial, which shows a 6 percent superior two-year survival and stroke rate when compared to surgical aortic valve replacement. Also the hemodynamics are superior.

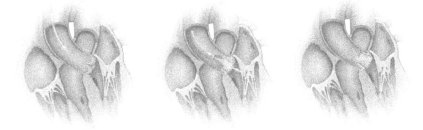

Figures courtesy of Fogarty Center

LESSONS LEARNED FROM DR. FOGARTY

- Dr. Fogarty decided to become a surgical inventor at the outset of his career and was met with early success showing thereafter the value of being committed to being an inventor.

- Early experiences with practical skills such as fly tying can be of pivotal value when the budding inventor needs to produce low-cost proof-of-concept prototypes.

- The emergence of a mentor at an early stage can empower the inventor and accelerate progress. The mentor will substantially influence the direction of the inventor's career. Dr. Jack Cranley believed in Fogarty's potential from an early stage and is given great credit by the inventor. Opportunities are presented when the inventor associates with young people who are set to strive in the future. The inventor has a duty to try diligently to adopt those of great promise and enthusiasm and provide encouragement.

- The career that starts early has a long runway when the true goal is to make a creative contribution. The message to young physicians is clear: begin to dream early and get a mentor or mentors for guidance.

- Dr. Dunfy probably prevented rapid progress by not authorizing Fogarty to work closely again with Dotter.

- The team that accumulates around a person with enthusiasm is essential to produce the momentum and exchange of ideas that accelerate an inventive process.

- The growth of a successful career leads you to mentor and teach aspiring young inventors. The benefit of being among those with energy and enthusiasm is career changing.

- People do not perform at full potential until they engage passionately in a compelling mission.

- Great people learn skills that allow them to flourish in any direction, as seen in Dr. Fogarty's new passion for prize-winning winemaking in the Napa Valley.

- The contributions of Dr. Fogarty's younger followers greatly expanded his own contribution, as can be seen by the careers of Dr. Fred Moll and Dr. Al Chin.

- Regional power and influence often become evident as synergy begins to cross-fertilize ideas.

- Dr. Fogarty has founded some 40 medical product companies and was inducted in 2001 into the National Inventors Hall of Fame.

- The combined effect of the regulatory burden and the need to qualify a product for "reimbursement" from insurers is the delay of product introduction by as much as seven years. Dr. Fogarty is passionate about trying to solve this issue in consultation with the FDA.

DR. JAMES HELLIWELL: START WITH A SIMPLE NEED

James Helliwell, a graduate of the UBC medical school, wished to improve the efficiency, availability, and safety of existing drugs. He built his career at St. Paul's Hospital in Vancouver, a hospital specializing in cardiology and cardiac surgery. Dr. Helliwell's family is notable because his father was a very influential academic economist from UBC. Dr. John Helliwell was senior fellow and codirector of the Canadian Institute for Advanced Research (CIFAR), which advises the Canadian government. He was the founder of the concept of social capital or happiness index. Hospital operating rooms are key centers of cost and value creation that are often wanting in efficiency. Dr. Helliwell developed systems that dramatically improved the delivery of services in the operating theatres. He did this by focusing on maximizing people's best skills, enhancing communication, and making the system more efficient while maintaining or increasing quality. This organizational bent was another example of his ability to study an area and apply rational solutions while he was carrying out a full workload in cardiac anaesthesia.

Dr. Helliwell suffered a sudden life-threatening health crisis that led to months in bed. While there, he asked himself, "If I cannot practice as a cardiac anaesthesiologist, is there a way I can solve problems and help make the world a better and healthier place?" He created Eupraxia Pharmaceuticals to achieve that goal. Anaesthesiology is all about planning for success or for failure. From his bed, he began querying the business world around him, trying to learn what caused similarly minded ventures to succeed and fail. This lead to the discovery of several risk commonalities across failures.

It was also important to him to ensure that success meant the greatest good for the greatest number of patients. With that, he focused on the treatment of osteoarthritis and pain.

Dr. Helliwell was unimpressed with the variability of drug kinetics in clinical medicine. To have a drug last a long time, you had to give far more than you wanted, leading to side effects. To get drugs to one part of the body, the high doses needed often target other tissues, producing collateral damage. For example, for arthritis, you want to treat the painful joint, not the rest of the body. His interest in this area led to a meeting with Dr. Tom Smith, a retired Harvard ophthalmologist with a long history in ophthalmic drug delivery innovation. Starting with a license from Dr. Smith's early technology, and a specific goal of delivering a drug in an ideal way, the Eupraxia scientific team built something new that delivered results going beyond their expectations. This mission was what is called a SMART goal: specific, measurable, achievable, relevant, and timely. To evaluate this goal, look at market size to understand the potential revenue.

Q. How many people have large-joint painful arthritis?

A. A third of all Americans, for a start.

Q. How many people have chronic pain requiring steroid injections?

A. Tens of millions in the United States alone, every year.

Dr. Helliwell's story is instructive from many points of view. Firstly, the acquisition of technology and specialized expertise allowed him to bypass a decade in a lab. This is an effective way to get a quick start and mimics the outstanding work of Victoria-based Aspreva Pharmaceuticals a decade earlier when the company developed CellCept for *Lupus erythematosis*. The company licensed the platform for very specific indications from Hoffmann-La Roche, which was selling the same drug in the transplant market. Following the success of developing CellCept, an application for the maintenance treatment of *Lupus erythematosis*, Aspreva, was sold to Galenica Holdings, a Swiss drug wholesaler, for US$980 million.

Assessing a business opportunity with the wide market scope seen by Eupraxia encourages investors and physicians. The Helliwell team has done a good job identifying markets. The job now is to prove the safety and effectiveness of the platform with use of steroids already on the market. After that, Eupraxia will demonstrate that troublesome systemic effects vanish and local drug delivery is extended for six or more months.

The board of Eupraxia is composed of seasoned local financial and business leaders with excellent credentials. The ability of Dr. Helliwell to recruit a strong board is a credit to the clearly defined value statement in the business plan. Dr. Amanda Malone received a master's degree in mechanical engineering from Stanford University and was the inaugural PhD student in Stanford's bioengineering department. Helliwell recognized in Dr. Malone a highly intelligent, creative, and dynamic scientist who was well suited to lead the development of such a disruptive program. Broad vision was the key in building the science and the company.

The second lesson is in the financial area. By being extremely capital efficient and maximizing non-dilutive government grants while staying focused on the goals required for the program to succeed, the company has pleased investors. The initial investor pool has been supportive of each round as each round has met its milestones and budget. The funds raised correspond well with money needed to advance the science to "clearly defined value inflection points," as James calls them. Funds are used in a very frugal manner that is lean on personnel and general expenditure. The self-restraint shown by management preserves more equity for early investors. The company is kept lean by outsourcing key research and testing.

LESSONS LEARNED FROM EUPRAXIA

- Establish a *large market opportunity* or a project that provides a platform technology into expanding markets over the life of the invention. Develop a business model that will suit the need.

- Investors will be loyal and supportive in subsequent rounds of financing if the benchmarks of progress are carefully set and achieved.

- Frugality in periods of lower activity preserves shareholder equity.

- Choose a mission that you can be passionate about.

- The strategy of licensing a portion of the IP for the activity spectrum of a drug or drug potentiator can be an excellent business strategy if the medical benefit includes a large market segment.

- Medical specialists must be creative in this new age when medical specialty boundaries are being redefined continuously. Those who do not find a way of adding value in their workplace may become redundant over time.

- The establishment of a powerful board is dependent on a compelling value statement in the business plan. There should be no mystery about how the company is going to succeed.

DR. AL CHIN: HOW TO INNOVATE

The potential of beginning early in life with a decision to become an inventor is shown by the career of surgeon inventor Dr. Al Chin. Dr. Chin started with biomedical engineering basic training at MIT, followed by a master's degree from Stanford. Deciding to study medicine, he earned an MD from the University of California, San Francisco, and entered surgical training at the University of Texas Parkland Hospital. Work with Dr. Thomas Fogarty resulted early on in many solid projects centered on catheter technology and vascular surgical instruments.

Origin Medsystems, Inc. was cofounded with Dr. Fred Moll. Origin perfected a series of products, including a laparo-lift device to allow gasless laparoscopy by manually lifting the abdominal wall. Another device, the spiral hernia tacker, permitted stapling of laparoscopic hernia patches through a 5 mm cannula rather than the standard 10 mm devices, which were state of the art at that time.

Origin Medsystems, Inc. included me in a focus group in the early 1990s. I went to Oakland for an Origin pig lab where spiral stapling prototypes were being tested. At that time, at lunch, I asked Dr. Chin what steps are needed to succeed as a surgeon inventor. He replied, "When you have an idea, it is imperative that you convert that idea to some form of physical test within one week." When this is done, two results are achieved:

1. The idea may be rejected or improved upon quickly, and
2. Most of the quality features of the idea will be learned by these simple means.

Dr. Chin subsequently became the vice president of research and development at Guidant Corporation when Origin was acquired by that company to become part of the cardiac surgery division. There was a period of legal conflict between Dr. Chin and Dr. Fogarty with respect to some aspect of their former collaboration. Dr. Fogarty regretted this, and after a period of difference, called Dr. Chin to have a peace lunch. This was followed by continued friendship and collaboration.

Pavilion was started in 2010 by Dr. Chin to continue his contributions to surgical innovation. Pavilion offers inventor services and extensive networks to aid the medical inventor. The skills acquired through years of successful exits are tacit knowledge that is retained by partners. These skills can be taught and brought to bear on new project ideas. The other benefit of this knowledge base is the ready assessment of the quality of the ideas prior to deep investment of time and money.

LESSONS LEARNED FROM DR. CHIN

- Do a simple prototype within one week to establish the validity of the idea. You will learn 90 percent of what you will ever know from this simple approach. Should the idea appear to work, serial prototyping should be done to enhance the understanding of possible benefits prior to raising or spending a lot of money. The information from this prototype can be added to the US provisional patent that you are creating.

- Begin your inventive career early in life.

- Teach young inventors.

DR. FREDRICK H. MOLL: INTUITIVE MEDICAL AND THE DA VINCI SURGERY SYSTEM

Dr. Fred Moll also decided early in his medical career to become an inventor after graduation from University of Washington's medical school with MD and MSc degrees. This is an example of early career commitment common to medical inventors.

Dr. Moll has been a serial innovator with an impressive track record following his early work cofounding Origin Medsystems. Subsequently, he has created a number of medical device companies and a successful venture fund, Hansen Partners.

The success of Origin and sale to Guidant set the two cofounders on divergent paths. Dr. Moll went on to collaborate on the development of the robotic da Vinci surgical system as well as many other projects extending Fogarty's contribution. The scale of the enterprise required to develop this advanced robotic system is impressive.

LESSONS LEARNED FROM DR. MOLL

- The decision to become a medical inventor was made at the outset of his career.

- Dream big or go home. Dr. Moll's BHAG was to develop the robotic da Vinci surgical system.

MACHAN/HUNTER: THE ANGIOTECH STORY

The Taxol stent was the first drug-eluting stent employed for treatment of cardiac atherosclerotic arterial disease. This invention, circa 1992, originated from an unlikely Vancouver site at UBC's Department of Surgery, Vascular Division, and from an unlikely team accidentally brought together. The story highlights the alertness and resourcefulness of some individuals and also the serendipitous nature of discovery.

The UBC Hospital's Department of Vascular Surgery led by Dr. Peter Fry was a small group of progressive surgeons who closely collaborated with interventional radiologists led by Dr. Lindsay Machan. On the fateful day, a medical student, Bill Hunter, was assigned to the service. Because of a shortage of interesting clinical material that day, Hunter was asked to make a scientific presentation of his choice. Hunter had recently served with the cancer treatment service of the Cancer Control Agency of British Columbia (CCABC) and decided to focus his presentation on the treatment of malignancy with the drug Taxol (paclitaxel), a local BC discovery that is isolated from the bark of the Pacific yew tree, *Taxus brevifolia,* and has proven to be an effective treatment for advanced breast cancer.

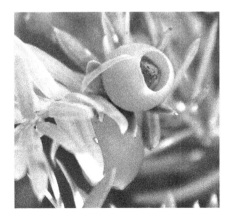

Taxol was of marginal interest to the vascular surgery group, but the presentation generated a discussion. Speculation began around the possibility of using Taxol's anti-angiogenesis effect for the vexing problem of tissue in-growth into bare metal stents. It is not clear how the idea developed during the discussion, but the combination of different backgrounds and different knowledge bases added depth to the discussion. Lindsay Machan, with his interventional radiology background, had intimate stent knowledge and was able to add high-level input. Bill Hunter was a keen student and became involved in the advancement of the idea along with Dr. Fry and Dr. Doyle.

The team developed considerable enthusiasm for this new idea because at that time there were no advanced projects adding drugs to stents and this seemed like a completely new area of research. The group was not primarily a research team, but the group members' inherent enthusiasm carried the day. They decided to take the idea further and study the potential by raising a friends-and-family round of investment of CAD $60,000 to begin development. An early provisional patent was placed in the US Patent and Trademark Office repository.

The team conceived a remarkable experiment to prove the utility of the idea. They used fertilized hens' eggs, which have a prominent, easily visualized microvasculature when the shell is partially removed. Chick chorioallantoic membrane (CAM) assays are readily examined with 160x magnification. The team selected four fertilized eggs and:

1. There was no treatment or intervention on the control egg.
2. Dilute Taxol solution was placed on the second egg.
3. Stent fragments were placed on the third egg.
4. Taxol and stent fragments were placed on the fourth egg.

The resulting development was then documented with serial microscopic photographs.

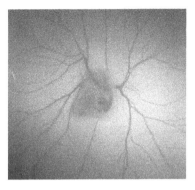

Fig. 14: Typical neo-vascuature growing on the surface of the chorioallantoic membrane of a hen's egg yolk.

This early work produced the expected result, which was that Taxol inhibited the growth of microvasculature, the stent material permitted growth of microvasculature, and the control egg grew as expected. When Taxol was combined with stent material, the microvasculature was again inhibited.

The pictures derived from this experiment, which cost approximately CAD 500, were subsequently used by Dr. Lindsey Machan's group to raise some CAD 450 million. The elegance of this experiment and its low cost show that clear thinking is the inventor's best ally. In the early stages of any inventive process, the inventor must find a way to prove the concept with the expenditure of as little money as possible. All too frequently, the new inventor becomes mesmerized by the details of the product and fails to understand the big-picture goal of enabling development of a company vehicle.

Often, the inventor thinks raising large sums of money is necessary to begin the awe-inspiring task of the development of the company. When such money is available, it distracts the team from the essence of product development or may be squandered on meaningless operational steps that don't really affect the value stream of the idea. Early deployment of large amounts of money on an inexperienced team is likely to lead to disaster. Focus on money raising and factors unrelated to the development of a real business are corrupting influences. Real business development focuses on getting a first effective product into the hands of a customer who is willing to pay a price that will produce profit. There is a right amount of financing for any given stage of company development. Insufficient funds will shock-stall the company at a critical time, destroying momentum and defeating the team. Excess money will surrender too much equity early and will disrupt product- and customer-centered growth. The balance is maintained by assuring that there is enough money to reach the next value inflection point where new investors will be able to appreciate recent company development.

This team, led by CEO Bill Hunter, carried out a rapid and effective execution to mature the product, which was then licensed to the newly created Angiotech.

At that time, there was no way to bind Taxol to the metal stent. The Taxol had to be released over an extended period of time to inhibit cell replication at the site of the stent. The chemical bonding, originally patented as a polymeric structure including Taxol as an example, was not limited to Taxol or even anticancer drugs. It offered potential attachment of a variety of heparinoids and other drugs. Slow delivery of the drug resulted in blood levels of Taxol 100 to 1000 times lower than those typically found during cancer chemotherapy.

The IP story began with the publication of US provisional patents on April 3, 1995; June 7, 1995; and July 19, 1993. They were useful in establishing a 1993 priority date. In 2001, these provisional patents were converted of to a series of full US patents, including compositions and methods for treating or preventing diseases of body passageways: US 6759431 B2. The inventors of the original patents are published as Lindsay S. Machan and William L. Hunter.

The basic idea of the provisional patent is to include as much detail as possible with pictures, graphs, experiments, and text to be drawn upon when the first real patent is written.

In the early years of Angiotech, the stewardship of MD/CEO Bob Hunter was outstanding. Angiotech became one of Vancouver's *Profit 100* magazine's fastest-growing companies. Revenue, a mere CAD 102,000 in 1994, had climbed in 1999 to CAD 4.4 million. In 1996, Hunter left his medical career to support the growth of the enterprise. Hunter qualifies as a genuine physician co-inventor able to transition into an entrepreneurial success.

Angiotech established a business relationship with Boston Scientific for stent sales and distribution and completed the arrangement with a US$14 million initial payment followed by a 1 percent royalty on certain sales. Boston Scientific was also given rights to sublicense the Angiotech technology to third parties. Boston Scientific, as a result of this acquisition and further scientific development, is a leader in coronary stent placement.

The fate of the two companies has been different since completion of this arrangement. Boston Scientific became a leader, even though the company suffered setbacks with recalls and the many risks associated with operating in this field. One of the recalls of more advanced Boston Scientific paclitaxel stents involved 100,000 stents and resulted in a dramatic loss in share value. The company remains a resilient and powerful player in this area. The fate of Angiotech, however, suffered from an inability to develop and commercialize any other blockbuster brand. The company sold its predominant assets, at which time the surgical product business had generated US$123 million while royalties generated US$15 million. Restructuring had occurred under court order in 2011. The revenue from the company sale was used to pay off corporate debt.

This story illustrates the challenge to successful companies who need to make a transition from a one-product company to a company that can sustain growth. There are two sources of such sustained growth: ideas originating from company inventors or ideas purchased outside the company. Many large companies rely entirely on mergers and acquisitions (M&A) activity to sustain growth, so there is a marketplace for companies and advanced products. The M&A skills for a champion team are rarely found in the start-up. The most skilled of these companies produce sustainable growth for many years and may have the stature of Johnson & Johnson over time. The single-product company often is fodder for growth rather than the source of a new rapidly growing enterprise.

Dr. William Hunter is now the CEO and director of Cardiome Pharma Corporation. The company has two cardiovascular products approved in Europe for treatment of recent onset atrial fibrillation (sold by Merck) and a treatment for acute coronary syndrome (tirofiban, marketed as Aggrastat).

Dr. Lindsay Machan made large contributions as cofounder of Angiotech and guided development of the company's products by being the high-level specialist at close range. Later, Dr. Machan chose to continue his career as an interventional radiologist and investor-mentor for aspiring young companies. Dr. Machan also made a pivotal contribution to the adoption of aortic stent products into vascular surgery practice in British Columbia.

The medical inventor must make a series of life decisions when assessing the options at each stage of company development. These are life-changing decisions. Withdrawal from active practice means ending a stage of life that has taken years of dedicated effort to achieve and offers security compared to the gyrations of a tech start-up company. Company leadership requires total commitment to give the start-up the best chance of survival.

LESSONS LEARNED FROM ANGIOTECH

- Serendipity can bring ideas together unexpectedly. An intelligent team can scrum around these ideas with effective action if the decision is taken promptly.

- Aggressive bootstrapping creates value rapidly on a modest budget if the idea is strong and novel.

- Execution creates value. The invention has great value, but most of the financial value harvested resides in the execution of the idea and making the sacrifices demanded by staying with the developing story. Inventors do not generally realize this because they reason that none of this would be possible without their great idea.

- The history of invention is littered with the carcasses of dead inventions that were not executed to extract the intrinsic value. Angiotech was an execution success story from the outset.

DR. GARY MICHELSON: A LESSON OF A DIFFERENT KIND

Perhaps the most highly rewarded inventor in the surgery space in recent years is Dr. Gary Michelson, an orthopaedic surgeon living in Los Angeles. Dr. Michelson developed numerous spinal implant devices, methods, and tools to assist the spinal surgeon. The impetus to begin this work was his grandmother, who suffered for years with spinal dysfunction pain and said to him, "You should become a doctor and solve this spine problem." This messaging was life changing.

The focus of Michelson's work coincided with the strategic needs of Medtronic for a new brand and technology in the growing field of spinal implant surgery. The plethora of Michelson patents, more than 900 in the end, coupled with an inventive new porous disc prosthesis, was licensed to Medtronic for a sum in the tens of millions, but a dispute developed. Medtronic considered some new ideas to be implicit in the old license, while Dr. Michelson was dissatisfied with the Medtronic lease performance. Medtronic sued, the inventor countersued, and the net result was that Medtronic was forced to pay US$1.3 billion in settlement. This whole saga was very controversial in the medical profession. Some believed that the ideas were public or created by others, but the fact remains that the Michelson legal team placed before the negotiators a strong parcel of facts that were endorsed by the court as the best way to resolve the IP dispute. The fundamental surgical contribution was a sustained value generator for patients and everyone associated.

LESSONS LEARNED FROM
DR. MICHELSON

- Patents give the inventor an opportunity for rewards based on the value of the contribution.

- While it is very fortunate to be able to link up with a great company, be on guard for any abuses that might come from this asymmetrical relationship.

- The early license agreement may result in an expensive legal battle that most inventors could never fund from their own resources.

- The intensity of the litigation activity is proportionate to the scale of any innovation market.

- Dr. Michelson is a prolific patent creator with a clever patent strategy.

- A compelling story of origin is helpful to market a personal brand.

PART TWO

IDEAS AND THEIR DEVELOPMENT

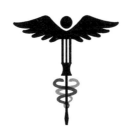

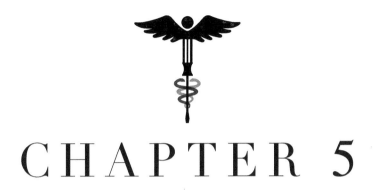

CHAPTER 5

THE MASTER PROBLEM LIST

The journey of a thousand miles begins with a single step.
—Laozi

Earlier in this book I touched on the value of being an inventor challenged by many possible ideas, as opposed to being the champion of a single creative solution. The danger posed by the single idea is that inventors or innovators become so enthralled that they expend time and energy promoting a concept that has no future in the market. Very often, those who have one favourite idea and lack the desire to explore other possibilities will actually avoid engaging in the systematic investigation that is necessary to establish market viability. Thus, instead of forging a dream into a reality, their reality, when focused on the wrong product, can become a nightmare.

I maintain, therefore, that it is important to avoid seeing yourself as the creator of an original idea that will amaze the world and that will lead to outstanding market success. Much better, particularly in the early stages, to adopt the attitude that you are a creative and inventive person who will consider many different problems, devise many potential solutions, evaluate and prototype often, and engage in the rigorous investigation necessary to determine acceptance and market viability. The belief that you can develop more than one idea will enable you to honestly critique and, if necessary, give up any unworthy line of investigation. You will own your ideas while preventing any specific idea from owning you. If you accept this philosophy of invention, you will need to create a list of problems based as much as possible on your own experience. The definition of the problem is the true starting point. Far too many innovative people have developed solutions based on their skill in a particular area of technology and then have wastefully spent months and years in search of applications for the work.

THE ROLE OF SERENDIPITY IN INVENTION

An invention may be a perfect solution for an unexpected pain point. Perhaps the best example of serendipity is the discovery of penicillin by Alexander Fleming who, in 1928, noticed that mould on his culture plates was preventing growth of his *Staphylococcus aureus* bacteria. The plates in his Imperial College lab were contaminated with a penicillium mould and exuded an antibacterial substance, which he called penicillin.

Remarkably, in 1897, a French scientist, Professor Ernest Duchesne, studied the competition between *E. coli* and *Penicillium glaucum*. His dissertation and publications were ignored by the Institute Pasteur. Duchesne was not able to bring this invention forward for whatever reason. This shows the necessity of being alert to the miracles that serendipitously appear from time to time.

ORDERLY DEVELOPMENT OF AN "IDEA LIST"

The problems you identify as worthy of solution may be listed in your personal or corporate "idea list." Include anything that you can imagine with your personal knowledge base without prejudgment. From your practice of medicine you will recall your biggest challenges or your daily aggravations. Ask yourself, "What if I were able to solve these problems?" The list will include general problems, such as cancer or diabetes, and specific technical issues, such as your unfulfilled dream of creating an image-guided, minimally invasive method for inguinal hernia repair.

A very long list may be achieved that will, by its existence, focus your thoughts on the problems and potential solutions. Some ideas will create more interest than others, depending on how much pain and anguish is generated by the problem. Truly vexing problems generate many solutions. In general, if there is great debate about the solutions currently available, the problem is not definitively solved but is still waiting for the ideal solution to come along. The search for solutions serves to alert you that this problem is worthy of effort. The corollary of this is that should you be brilliant and find a practical solution that is easy to learn, easy to apply, and effective, your solution will likely be adopted. The contemplation of problems on such a list can generate early ideas that might lead to unique solutions.

THE BLUE OCEAN STRATEGY

The notion of the blue ocean is useful for those trying to deal with new ideas by helping them decide where to focus their creative efforts.

Ideas in the blue ocean concept are divided into two categories. The first path is termed the blue ocean strategy path, which describes the wide blue sea where there is nothing to hinder your passage. The blue ocean zone in business is an open area where you can operate freely because it is fresh, new, and devoid of competition, a monopoly. The second of these paths, the red ocean strategy path, is by contrast a dangerous place where intense competitive activity lurks from established competitors.

In a red ocean you will be competing against existing commodity products and against large companies with entrenched dominance and great skill battling in the marketplace. The blue ocean space is a void where you may create a product where none exists and no market exists. You must create the product and then the market.

BLUE OCEAN OPPORTUNITY	RED OCEAN OPPORTUNITY
Creates an uncontested new monopoly	Competes in an existing busy market
Invention to solve an unsolved problem	Innovation on an old solution to add value
Competition is nonexistent	Competes against established powerful players
Creates a new customer set that did not exist	Fights for customers owned by others
Adds new value that commands higher price	Lower price to try to break into market
Company seeks differentiation and low COGs	Company battles with new features and low cost
Possibly a disruptive invention if practice changes	An improvement but no disruption occurs
Paradoxically starts with a small market	Starts attacking a large identified market

Fig. 15: Summary of the qualities of blue and red oceans.

This is the province of the disruptive innovator, someone who can quietly work unopposed and invisible, as Elizabeth Holmes did for ten years at Theranos to create a new set of customers in a new market. The GlideScope video laryngoscope and the LMA, both of which changed the airway management paradigm, illustrate this.

W. Chan Kim and Renée Mauborgne introduced this concept in a 2004 *Harvard Business Review* article wherein they described a wonderful Canadian example of the blue ocean concept created by Guy Laliberté of the Cirque du Soleil. This circus, founded in 1984, became a multinational success story based on reinventing the circus as an entertainment venue that approximates art in every aspect of its shows. When Cirque started to grow from Montreal, it had no competition. The differentiation from the Barnum & Bailey circus concept is clear. Cirque created demand in a space entirely different without ever competing against the classic circus venue featuring lion acts, elephant shows, and trapeze artists.

In *Blue Ocean Strategy* (Kim and Mauborgne, 2005), W. Chan Kim and Renee Mauborgne discuss six methods of reconstructing market boundaries to create blue ocean opportunities:

1. Looking across alternative industries at the way customer needs are satisfied. An example could be high-speed intercity travel needs that may be satisfied by commuter jet service or slower train and road transport. An example of train transport would be the conceptualization of a high-speed rail service that could compete on certain city pairings by reducing the inconvenience of getting to outlying airports and time spent going through security while losing some speed over the ground. The new service concept would create blue ocean customers, including those who have a fear of flying and who enjoy the relative luxury of high-speed rail service.

2. *Creation of a blue ocean product in the commodity undergarment space.* The conceptualization of Spanx is an example of taking a personal pain point and creating a product to address the new need, after which the inventor prototypes to find the best solution to this specific customer problem, as shown below.

The invention of Spanx is an interesting story of the creation of a blue ocean customer set that exploited several trends and needs in the market. The newly created affluent market is both aging and getting heavier. Sara Blakely graduated from Florida State University with a degree in communications and went from working at Disney World to selling fax machines. The personal pain of being unable to find pantyhose with seamless toes was her inspiration. She embarked on a series of experiments to modify existing products. At age 27, she invested her life savings of US$5,000 and moved to Atlanta to develop her own pantyhose concept. Bootstrap prototyping for one year led to a product with a custom waistband suited to customer girth, coupled with robust body-shaping support designed to replicate desirable body habitus for a portly, aging population. Her testing on family and friends allowed her to eliminate undesirable features and produce a comfortable patented product.

Blakely wrote the patent description herself:

> A pantyhose garment is provided that has relatively sheer leg portions that end with knitted-in welts just below or above the knees, and a reinforced control top portion having good shaping and control characteristics that terminate at the top of the waist region with a knitted-in welt. The pantyhose undergarment provides the user with shaping support, and because the lower leg is bare, it gives the user the freedom to wear any type of shoe (i.e., open-toed shoes, sandals, etc.).

Pantyhose worn with open-toed shoes are usually undesirable and also dangerous because the foot may slip in the shoe due to the lack of friction between the pantyhose and the shoe. In addition, there are many occasions when the user wants a more casual look in clothing, and therefore pantyhose on the foot and ankle would not be desired. The reinforced control top portion extends down the leg portions of the pantyhose far enough to provide support over the "saddlebag" and cellulite regions of the body. The knitted-in welt at the waist region blends into the control top without causing waist constriction. Similarly, the knitted-in welts at the ends of the leg portions blend into the leg portions without causing leg constriction. The overall design provides the user with a smooth, tight appearance when worn under clothing, without causing the user to suffer discomfort.

The name Spanx was also important in creating the product, which provided power to grow what is now a billion-dollar company. The above US patent description includes all that she learned from her extended personal and family prototyping activity. The benefits are clearly described. The success of the invention has proven that the user-friendly features were powerful. Sara noticed that strong brands often had a sharp K sound in their names—Kodak, Coca-Cola, Kindle—so she created the harsh-sounding, naughty word *Spanx* as her product name.

There is more to this story because Sarah realized the uniqueness and superiority of her sturdy support garments. No other underwear gave such excellent support and shapely body figure, even in the presence of excessive body fat. These qualities allowed creation of a new set of obese customers at a time when there is an obesity epidemic.

3. *Looking across the chain of buyers and producing a strategy that cuts out a target group to be addressed in a new way.* For example, Johnson & Johnson recently changed the target of one product when the company indirectly advertised to nurses rather than doctors by creating a "thank-you statement of appreciation for nurses."

4. *Looking across complementary product and service offerings to provide new services to couple with existing industries.* For example, you could provide designer meals for onboard consumption to compete with deteriorating service on global airlines. These could be sold near the departure lounges or for consumption in business-class lounges, and they could generate a scalable business.

5. *Looking across functional or emotional appeal to buyers.* Note: Saturn Biomedical Systems capitalized on elimination of "airway anxiety," the unspoken fear of loss of control with severe consequences, by giving a 99.9 percent certainty of a view of the airway for intubation success. The product was easily demonstrated to users, and by use of an intelligent group of key physicians and certified registered nurse anaesthetists (CRNAs), the word rapidly spread, creating a large new customer set.

6. *Looking across time and projecting trends into the future.* Note: To some extent, the Spanx example does this by focusing on the population-aging trend and also the obesity explosion.

CREATING THE NEW WORLD BY CHOOSING WHERE TO INNOVATE

Innovation that reproduces the old order is not innovation. The essence of converting a red ocean opportunity into a blue ocean one is to fully understand the needs of the marketplace and how existing products do not meet them. Think of the vast number of low-cost commodity coffee machines replicated and produced in the Far East for sale in our Big Box stores. The Nespresso business model is instructive. Machines are sold by many sellers to generate market base. The high-cost, high-value, high-profit coffee single-use capsules are sold only by Nespresso direct sales so that the primary profit source of the business is captured 100 percent. Customers get efficiency by not brewing excess coffee and convenience from the brewing speed. They are willing to pay a high price for the coffee brewer and pay a high price buying the coffee capsules in what ends up as a service cost.

Peter Drucker stated that the goal of business is to create a customer. Customers are created by developing a product people want to buy. Should you identify a value that the commodity products don't provide, then, by definition you will develop a blue ocean product. The inventive difference and the ability to protect the space by IP, trademarking, and rapid growth will define its significance. While this may sound obvious, it is of critical importance to understand these facts completely.

LESSONS LEARNED

- Competition is for losers: Whenever possible, create a monopoly by developing blue ocean products.

Monopolies are the enemy of price competition and therefore are opposed by government and consumer action groups.

- "The goal of business is to create a customer" (Drucker).

- "The unique customer is created by the unique product."

- Innovation that reproduces the old order is not innovation.

- William James said, "First, a new theory is attacked as absurd; then, it is admitted to be true but obvious and insignificant; finally, it is seen to be so important that its adversaries claim they themselves discovered it."

- Edward de Bono said, "Creative thinking is not a talent; it is a skill that can be learnt. It empowers people by adding strength to their natural abilities, which improves teamwork, productivity, and, where appropriate, profits."

- YouTube is a very rapid way of understanding processes and viewing content pertaining to your ideas. The learning acquired in this way can be added to the US provisional patent document, which gains value while you work and discover.

- Use Google Scholar to set up an automatic reporting search on your key topics.

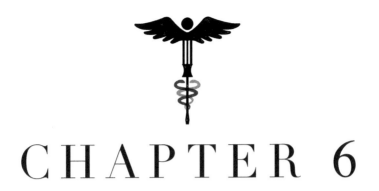

CHAPTER 6

INTELLECTUAL PROPERTY

The new inventor has serious anxiety-provoking questions to answer. How much to reveal? To whom? How? With what protection? The first principle is that you disclose only on a need-to-know basis. There must be a good business reason to tell anyone what you are thinking. Others can and will occasionally be in a position to exploit this knowledge. Don't make a public disclosure at a meeting, at a professional gathering, or any public venue. There is little benefit and some real risk that the idea will be rendered unprotected. When presenting to individuals and small groups, nondisclosure agreements must be in place so that persons present cannot claim that a public unprotected disclosure occurred. Once the patent is in place, you can discuss its content and implications, but keep in mind that extensions of the IP are essentially new IP and must be protected by nondisclosure. The need-to-know rule is the safest way to proceed.

Intellectual property knowledge is also a key asset, and reading patents is the best way to start to understand. Reliance on professionals is best practiced when you have a total grasp of the decisions being made and why they are chosen. Patents are a huge storehouse of specific area knowledge and can reveal what solutions are currently known. There is no point in inventing something that was patented years before, unless you can make a significant advancement in the art. Google Patent, the European Patent Office, and the US Patent and Trademark Office are searchable sites and will provide much information to the inventor. Searching these sources is a skill and duty for the manager of ideas. Should you fail to detect relevant patents and potential conflicts, time and money will be lost. There is also a risk that you could end up in a patent contest when the fledgling company is small and weak. Generally, a patent battle will cost US$1 million to begin with and could quickly get to US$5 million or much more. This should be avoided for the small company, even though a granted patent might be considered the entry ticket for such a contest.

The history of Dr. Gary Michelson, however, shows what a sharp-witted and persistent inventor can achieve. Fortunately, the funds to fight were, in part, provided by the earlier settlements that he and his company had obtained.

Early in the process a preliminary "freedom to practice" study done by a legal expert will show if there is obvious potential to wilfully encroach on others patents. Specify the limits of your budget so that expenses don't run out of control. Prioritization is critical to move the tasks forward in a sequence that matures the project and increases value with affordable expenditure.

Professional help is essential, but there are simple things you can do yourself, such as filing multiple US provisional patents around the idea and its details. If your experimental work on the invention is accurately described, you must get a professional to coalesce the knowledge into a formal patent application within one year. Should the claims be accepted, the 17-year clock will start ticking until expiry of the primary patent. The cost of a patent application of average complexity might be in the US$10,000 range, but this is only the beginning of a long train of fees and maintenance.

The field of intellectual property is complex and filled with nuance. Some have likened it to real estate, where property is defined and claimed to be discrete from that around it, but concepts are less concrete. Patent applications claim inventiveness and uniqueness. The submitted patent application is examined by patent office specialists, who judge whether the application is new art or has been previously thought of. Intellectual property includes the patent portfolio combined with all of the steps required to convert the patents into a salable product. Because learning is continuous, the current product will usually exhibit nuances that depart from the patents held. This process must be reviewed regularly to create new applications as required to fully cover the cleverness of your ongoing work.

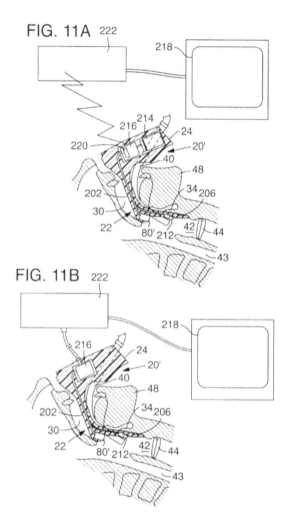

Fig. 16: These images from the GlideScope patent drawings show both a wired option and a wireless option. The early patents also show a variable angle device that can range from 5 to 85 degrees depending on the needs of the airway geometry. This option allows a full spectrum of viewing from direct laryngoscopy to highly angled laryngoscopy, using one device. The GlideScope

patents I filed were US 6,142,144; US 6,655,377; US 6,543,447; and European patent 1307131.

FIRST TO INVENT

The older first-to-invent concept allowed the inventor to submit dated documents that proved that initial work on the invention occurred at a place and time that would become a date of invention. This practice was dropped by Canada in 1989, the Philippines in 1998, and the USA on March 16, 2013.

FIRST TO FILE

The first-to-file concept was adopted in Canada and the Philippines as a new concept. This does not require the filer to be the inventor but, rather, the first to apply to the patent office to obtain recognition as the patent owner.

FIRST INVENTOR TO FILE

This concept, adopted in the USA in 2011 and in force since March 16, 2013, attributes the patent to the first inventor to file and takes away the right of inventors to submit evidence of prior invention documented privately. The publication of an idea prior to a formal patent application could prevent an inventor from getting a patent because the inventor has, in effect, donated the idea to the world. The new US law is controversial because it raises constitutional concerns.

THE UNIQUE IDEA

To patent an idea, it must be unique. The test for uniqueness is that the idea must be both novel and inventive. The invention must not have existed before.

Novelty means the idea must not be present in recorded literature or in fields of work. The patent office will endeavour to search the major databases of the US Patent and Trademark Office, the European Patent Office, public forums, and other major databases to see if the ideas in the new patent have shown up previously.

The idea is inventive if skilled workers could not achieve the result delivered by the product by simply using their normal trade skills and supplies to adjust the work path. In short, workers would not be able to craft your product by using the usual methods but, rather, only by taking the clever, inventive steps that you have provided.

Uniqueness is not as simple as it sounds in a world of millions of ideas. You must make a judgment and take yet another risk. The problem is complicated by the crossover that may occur when a principle is applied in another field of work and escapes the notice of patent applicants.

The method patent for the invention of cold fusion, for example, could define the way to produce sustained fusion. The patent applicants would thus own the right to exploit the process. Workers could not do this using established methods.

The device patent of the marine sextant, for example, had it never been conceived before, would be allowed because of the detailed method of celestial navigation embodied in the device.

Methods and devices are thus patentable. New inventors must explore patents and understand them with little or no formal training. The answer, once again, is to begin by reading patents and becoming familiar with the form, content, and subject matter of the inventive field. The logic will slowly become apparent to the inventor, who will see how others have tried to solve the problems. This is an indispensible learning step. Discussions with a professional patent attorney will continue the education process and lead to more correct decisions. The US Patent and Trademark Office offers inventors many education services that describe steps to be taken during and after a search. Assistance in crafting a US provisional patent may establish a priority date for the inventor, which starts the 17-year patent clock running and signals the beginning of protection.

The method I believe to be efficient and practical for the new inventor is to begin writing a US provisional patent application early in the study of the new idea. This process begins with a trial concept of the patent name. What is the device or method in short form? What is the date? Who is the inventor or inventors? What references to prior patents are close to this idea?

The strength of the patent position will have a great influence on the final price your company will command years later. The expenditure of money early to establish patent coverage will not be wasted but will give the best chance for a profitable exit for the founders and early investors.

PATENT CLAIM WRITING IS A HIGH ART

The first independent claim on a patent is as general as possible so that the principle can achieve broad coverage. The standard filing fee for a utility application with the US Patent and Trademark Office covers up to three independent claims and up to 20 total claims before additional filing fees are incurred. Adding independent claims adds cost at all levels, domestic and foreign. The patent office may take excess independent claims and demand that you file several separate patents to cover different inventions. The dependent claims relate to the independent claims to add detail or color to the claim and bring in specific features that will also be protected. The most powerful patent needs a clear, broad, strong dominant idea that is essential to practice the invention.

THE NONDISCLOSURE AGREEMENT

Most inventors fret about secrecy, believing that even the barber will steal the idea, whereas the world really doesn't want to know you or your idea until it has dented someone's stable earning stream. When this happens, IP is extremely important for you and the enterprise that wants to take it into the future. Therefore, you must *only* discuss the project when you need to share information for concrete business reasons. When you do share, it must be under the cover of a nondisclosure agreement.

Public expression of the idea without protection is the equivalent of donating the idea to the world. Professional guidance should be taken as soon as possible. File new IP at every opportunity to build a virtual picket fence around your core IP. This will make it risky for encroachers, as complexity requires lawyers to make a call that has a risk of error. Lawyers are risk averse and may, to be conservative, recommend avoiding your picket fence. The entrepreneur's specialty is taking risk after risk and surviving to tell the tale, but intellectual property is not the place to take risk.

THE GRANTED PATENT: THE RIGHT TO SUE

A patent is granted by a sovereign state to practice the teachings of the invention for 17 to 20 years provided the patent holder pays the required periodic fees. The patent subject domain may be extended by application for a continuation, in part, in the country of original prosecution. Rights in foreign countries are obtained by selecting a range of geographies included in the protection. The Patent Cooperation Treaty covers this area of international law.

There is often overlap between ideas and patents granted, not unlike North American native land claims in which different groups often seek recognition of traditional ownership of the same geographic area. This legal territory is tested in court to define the patent boundaries. Generally, the legal activity grows with the financial dimensions of the business. New players enter by defining their turf with a differentiation nuance that claims to make their device patentable. The battle intensifies as the market dollar value increases. Would-be competitors increasingly try to break into the space.

The holder of a granted patent has the right to defend the patent in a court challenge or may pursue an apparent infringer. The infringer may try to find evidence that the patent has been compromised by prior disclosure of the idea. The legal fees for attempting to defend patent claims start in the region of US$1 million. This number tends to grow because the complexity of the battle depends, in part, on the financial strength of your opponent. Powerful companies have sufficient strength to wear down a small company or individual, with the result that the rights are weakened or lost. This must be considered when purchasing a small company or its patent position. The benefits of winning patent battles may be substantial, especially in the USA where wilful exploitation of someone else's patent claims can lead to triple damages. The damages are defined by demonstrated loss of market share, profitability, costs associated with the battle, and losses. Major collateral damage is caused by distraction of the management team from the passionate tasks of company building.

Companies have been created for the sole purpose of doing battle for an inventor thought to have a strong prospect of winning in court. These companies take value from the settlement to compensate for their high risk. This helps the inventor with a strong position but no money to fight.

A very dangerous group of patent trolls purchase IP with the goal of attacking companies large and small to try to force an agreement that will give them revenue or dominance. Regulators are looking at developing constitutionally acceptable legislation to limit this practice because the effect is to destroy smaller companies and cause distracting expensive litigation for larger entities. An example this strategy is Blackberry's victimization by the patent-holding company NTP in a contest over e-mail software. Blackberry maintained that in-house software invalidated the patents purchased by NTP from inventors, but the court found that this was not true. The protracted battle was ultimately settled with payment of $612.5 million by Blackberry.

PROTOTYPING FOR PRODUCT UTILITY

The development of a sophisticated product development process (PDP) is the ultimate need of a technology-based company. In the beginning this is rendered down to a series of simple important steps leading to selection of the most promising ideas.

Generation of a blue ocean opportunity in a world of red oceans requires a product that will create customers. Exploiting the ideas from your product funnel, the "new product idea list," will give you your start. You must validate each idea on the list by following the recommendation of Dr. Al Chin to create a simple functional prototype to do the initial assessment of the product concept.

You must then ask the questions:

1. How large is the potential market?
2. How would we be able to develop this market with our resources?
3. How can this be made and sold with margins that make it a profitable business?

Prototyping your way to functionality is a continuous process of refinement. The inventors featured in this book are all aggressive prototypers. The power of prototypes is illustrated in the book *Experimentation Matters: Unlocking the Potential of New Technologies for Innovation* by Stefan H. Thomke (Thomke, 2003). The book describes New Zealand's defense of the America's Cup race. This example demonstrated the utility of prototyping relentlessly to approximate perfection in design.

The American team touted their access to the General Dynamics Electric Boat submarine-design wave tank as a valuable asset for design of the US challenger's hull. Resources from Boeing's computer-based simulation equipment were available.

The New Zealand team did a more low-cost approach using serial modifications to the boats, followed by sailing each design change in the waters where the race would take place, with the actual crew and the local winds. The New Zealand yacht *Black Magic NZL 60* went on to win the America's Cup in 2000. The New Zealand 2000 syndicate achieved its victory largely through serial prototyping. Serial prototyping can be more or less costly and time consuming compared to computer-aided design, depending on the circumstances.

Computer-aided design is relied on universally now because the number of variants that can be vetted for testing is greatly increased. A distillate of these can be used for the final prototyping to perfect the design. The Parametric Technology Corporation product Pro/ENGINEER is a commonly used design modeling software. The final designs are tested in real conditions, where effects are seen that were not appreciated when the computer programming was done. Discovery is common when real objects are tested in the real world. The ideal is to get the easy learning done by simulations in a cost-effective manner and then begin another phase of learning in the real world. If the thinking is powerful and the simulation is cleverly designed, the product can move very efficiently to a stage of perfection.

DELIVERING VALUE BY PROTOTYPING

- Serial prototyping is a method whereby each prototype is completed, studied, and altered. The problem with this method is the possible occurrence of "functional fixation" whereby you become design limited by your first attempt.
- Prototyping will cost more than you think and will take much longer than you can imagine because each embodiment must be made to a verified and validated market-ready stage before human tests can be done. Subsequent changes must be fully documented by an

approved change process leading to new approvals and extensions of the protocol.

- Parallel prototyping is an approach in which numerous approaches are built as competing designs. This method allows more options to be developed and is usually done early in the process of design selection.

- The value of knowledge base and training in another field away from the field of invention is huge. Cross-training in engineering and anaesthesia offers a good example of a fertile combination that may lead to unexpected, unique value.

DESIGN REQUIREMENT LIST: SET EASILY VERIFIED AND VALIDATED PRODUCT GOALS

When you have established that the original idea has utility in solving the clinical problem, the next step is to describe a lean set of goals to begin the conversion to a product that can be manufactured reliably.

Begin with a detailed description of the task the invention is expected to solve. The next step is to write a draft of the design requirements that the proposed product will need to carry out the mission. This list can be converted into exact engineering specifications.

Specifications are goals the engineers focus on to build a product prototype that can be tested. The cost of verification of specifications and validation of design requirements leading to efficacy demands that these requirements be kept to the essentials. Control is essential because if you have 50 requirements, each will need costly testing that repeats with each product modification.

> *There is surely nothing quite so useless as doing with*
> *great efficiency what should not be done at all.*
> —Peter Drucker

THE COMPANY SHALL BE COMPLIANT

The compliance commitment must be incorporated into the vision statement of the company as a core value. Noncompliance or partial compliance is a bad business strategy that introduces legal and operational vulnerability. Compliance is expensive for the start-up, and perfection is rare, but the process needs a top priority.

Verification will assure that specifications have been met. Validation that the product actually completes the mission for the user with safety and efficacy must be done. Failure to make the product easy to use and learn will result in slow adoption, which could kill the fledgling company. The product must extend the capabilities of the user.

Also:

1. Goals to cover use in cold-weather operation, device abuse, user neglect of the device, and extended use must be created.

2. How many times will the device be used over its expected life, and how will it fail? Does the failure of the device allow for a plan B to be safely carried out, or is

redundancy necessary?

3. Regulatory submissions will need to account for the usual and the unexpected use cases so that a planned failure mode is avoided.

The medical device standard is the International Organization for Standardization (ISO) 13485 qualification, which is audited by independent auditors such as TUV. The Underwriters Laboratories (UL) and Canadian Standards Association (CSA) minimum safety requirements are essential as baseline safety testing and will be matched by good manufacturing practices (GMP).

THE OPEN INNOVATION CONCEPT

Henry Chesbrough, executive director of the Center for Open Innovation at the University of California's Haas School of Business created the "open innovation" concept of ideas and IP as existing in a pool where inventive concepts co-exist with external concepts that provide knowledge to be mined for usable ideas. This replaces the classic Bell Labs concept of a fortress of ideas and IP, protected in a company idea vault to be used and protected only by the company.

Looking outward toward a world of ideas, you can delve into all the existent ideas and build a collage of collaboration with others' ideas, for a price. The company may blend inventions into an innovative system of greater value than that created by one isolated invention.

The open innovation concept has benefits and faults. Purchase of ideas or companies to satisfy overall strategic goals is now common.

Development of ideas in-house has been found to be challenging and requires team members who are skilled and focused on invention.

OPEN INNOVATION ADVANTAGES

- The innovative process gains advantage from many thinkers.
- External idea use may be cost-effective and flexible.
- Collaboration with customers on ideas requires that the ownership of new IP resulting from the custom designs resides with your company.
- Synergy can be identified between internal and external IP to produce a complex solution.

OPEN INNOVATION DISADVANTAGES

- Interacting with others can lead to compromised confidentiality.
- Loss of competitive advantage may occur by alerting others to your direction.
- It may be difficult to decide who owns what.
- Legal battles may ensue if the collaboration is not well designed and defined by contract before the work begins.
- Controlling people and resources from two entities is complex.
- Purchase of IP may be the simplest approach.

LESSONS LEARNED

- Explore the educational resources of the US Patent and Trademark Office and become skilled at patent reading.

- Use the US provisional patent format as a repository of knowledge as you learn about the place of your idea in the "sea of ideas."

PART
THREE

BUILDING A COMPANY

Lesson: *Competition Is for Losers; Create a Monopoly*

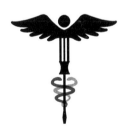

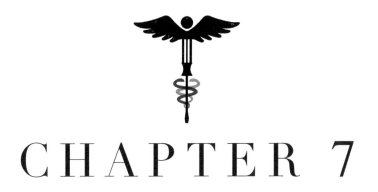

CHAPTER 7

THE BIG PICTURE

As an inventor, you create a prototype, and then, as an entrepreneur, you embark on a project to build a company to complete the design and build a product. You must realize at the very beginning that the company is being built over a period—it could be as long as ten years—before it is sold. The ownership of the company should be closely held by founders and should only be surrendered as a last resort to raise money for start-up and growth. Generally, use your own and family money combined with sweat equity to define the initial product. Bootstrap as long and as far as possible without selling shares so that you are working mainly for your own benefit, creating the initial value. Be certain at an early stage that your partners agree on methods that facilitate exit, for reasons that will develop over time. Typically, relationships and work contributions are asymmetrical, and equity should reflect this. Shotgun clauses or other understandings are, ideally, agreed upon early in partnerships. The last thing you want is to arrive at a sale, in the future, in which someone's widow or family fails to agree to the sale and prevents a clean exit. Discuss this with your legal representative at the outset.

THE CHANGING ROLE OF THE COMPANY

Modern concepts define two kinds of companies that are fundamentally different. The first kind is the *perfect competitor* that, by virtue of its culture and approach to customer satisfaction, innovates a steady value stream that stays ahead of the competition. The second kind is the *inventive company*, which abhors competition. These kinds of companies have products that are so different that there are no competitors. These rare companies have become much more prevalent because of the digital revolution, which, like the historic Industrial Revolution, is based on increased efficiency. The earlier revolution replaced hand labour with machines, whereas the digital revolution replaces hand labour with digital processes. The new era of digital progress has led to many ideas, such as PayPal, Google, Digital Banking, Apple Ecosystem, and FaceTime.

The new digital giants have been able to entrain capital and become *virtual monopolies* with wide public adoption of the platform. The total amount of monetary value created is huge because monopoly creates sustained growth of revenue and profit. Monopolies are under continuous pressure from government regulators who abhor the concentration of power and lack of choice. These new market leaders argue that they are not monopolistic by redefining the market concept. For example, Google is a monopolistic search engine but defensively claims its real market is advertising.

Earlier monopolies were vertically integrated giants of value creation. The Canadian Pacific Railway (CPR) in Canada, for example, was encouraged to span the country with its rail line by being given 20 miles of property on each side of the track. The railroad used that land to build a chain of premium resort properties across the country and spawn an international breadbasket grain industry serviced by CPR trains. This old method of creating monopoly could only be done with a well-executed great vision (BHAG). We must bear this in mind because value creation and value collection by innovators today remains optimized by the monopoly concept. The ordinary company must create value by innovating without benefit of monopoly.

The Microsoft Windows example is instructive. The dominance of the Windows operating system and Internet Explorer was attacked for more than ten years by the US Government and the European Union in the belief that these systems would dominate for the foreseeable future. They were hobbled by constant attack. What could not be foreseen was that the Android operating system (OS), sponsored by Google and Samsung, was about to become the dominant mobile OS leaving Windows a distant second. Apple has developed the dominant ecosystem for the moment. These massive shifts in the market should discourage governments from trying to predict the future and interfere with dynamic market forces.

COMPANY BASICS THAT MATTER

The start-up company is a temporary entity whose task is to define a viable product and create a profitable business model. The company grows in complexity as follows:

THE START: 1-19 EMPLOYEES. FOCUS ON THE PRODUCT AND REFINE THE BUSINESS MODEL.

The start-up has every possible risk. Like an onion, the progressive layers of risk need to be peeled away. Early risks include:

1) start-up risk: will it go at all?
2) founder risk: can the founders become skilled leaders?
3) product development risk: can founders make a product that works?

Lessons to be learned:

1. In the beginning, it is you and your idea. Make and test a proof of concept prototype.
2. This is the provisional US patent year; prototyping adds features.
3. Avoid hiring, save money, and use contractors.
4. Bootstrap the company and the product to satisfy one customer completely.
5. Start a chart of accounts to refine the business model by use of the "Business Model Canvas" nine areas defined by Alexander Osterwalder.

MANAGEMENT BEGINS: 20-49 EMPLOYEES

Develop a simple, clearly defined reporting structure that places employees into roles on an organization chart. Clarity and transparency are key so that everyone has a single person to report to. Dotted lines and other similar reporting paths cause confusion, anxiety, and conflict. Political activities are a symptom that the organization chart is flawed or people are losing efficiency to anxiety or confusion. The solution to this problem is transparency and enforcing the structure while building alignment.

The product will mature, and launch targets will emerge. Developing culture to produce team alignment is critical. At this time, the rhythm begins to emerge, powered by a metronome effect (discussed later).

- Daily stand-up meetings of key groups, lasting 15 minutes every morning, are organized to answer the question, why are we paying you today? The meeting is not for problem solving but for cross-communication leading to alignment.
- Weekly meetings, in contrast, allow in-depth discussion of issues and solutions.
- Monthly lunches or all-hands meetings allow management to repeatedly focus company attention on key goals and key alignment issues.
- Growth risk: Company systems must be mature and culture must be scalable at this point. Enhance the business model.

CONTINUED GROWTH PHASE: 50+ EMPLOYEES

Complexity increases exponentially as the number of people increases. Systems that are scalable, written down, and accessible are the key to cultural strength. Leaders must refine culture so that the employees are still aligned with management goals. Employee wikis can be used to record how you want things done and why. Experienced executives will be needed to produce accelerated growth. HR is a vital component at this juncture as the number of special-skill people increases. Quality HR enables employee growth and produces salary range bands that provide order. Always remember the quality of your hires determines success or failure of the business. The CEO must trust managers and be free to spend time on business strategy and business development. Develop a culture where direct reports prepare presentations and plans to present to superiors taking responsibility for themselves and those under them. Thus, managers can review plans and approve with need for only minor suggestions. This allows leaders to perform higher-level tasks.

THE PRODUCT AS AN ENGINE OF COMPANY GROWTH

The first product is an opportunity to build a company; it is not an end in itself. The initial offering is a platform for innovation and exploration. The physician inventor may believe that the "exciting new invention" is the real product, but, in the end, a product is but one element of the successful company. Inventor skills are vital, but most of the value creation occurs when the "execution phase" creates and delivers a real product. Those who stay with the company through this phase will garner greater rewards as the revenue begins to accumulate.

The physician inventor is not likely to have much ability for business leadership. The physician has highly focused training that will be of such intensity as to allow little time for business thoughts. Business skills are acquired by diligent study and application to the tasks of the business. The following topics will be important to the growth of an entrepreneur.

GEOFFREY MOORE: THE TECHNOLOGY ADOPTION CURVE AND THE CHASM

The product is expected to power the growth of the company and will do this if it has what is called the killer application to provide a solution to a vexing problem that causes pain in the market. A powerful product linked to an excellent business plan will follow the adoption curve described by Moore in his book *Crossing the Chasm*. This monumental work describes the path of a product brought into the market with enough energy to succeed. Moore's adoption curve places a gap in the adoption trajectory he calls the "valley of death" or "chasm," which describes the transition from the enthusiasm of the visionaries and early adopters to the early majority customers.

The technology enthusiasts or innovators are dream seekers who are not afraid of failure, love adventure, and are respected by each other but doubted by the masses. Many will call them lunatics. Working together with the new company, they will introduce the opportunity to everyone. The visionary group loves the new idea's potential to produce disruptive change and is willing to ignore or minimize the shortcomings of the product. This group drives change.

Visionary early adopters are poised to become the evangelists who will lead their peers to the idea. Visionaries eventually become recognized and trusted by their peers. The information gathered from the technology enthusiasts and visionaries can be used to upgrade the product so that when selling to the early majority, the experience is as full and exciting.

The visionaries and the company lead the product across the valley of death or chasm. The inspiration causes pragmatists to begin acquiring the product and its concept.

The early majority are real mainstream pragmatic consumers who want a fully featured product that works as expected and has few glitches when used on a protracted basis. This group waits until there is acceptance from the visionaries in the field so that they and their patients will be free of risk.

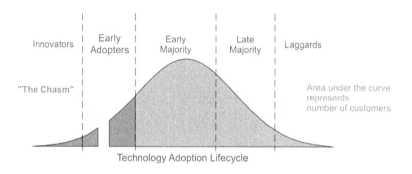

Fig. 17: The adoption curve and chasm of Geoffrey Moore.

The late majority conservatives hold back until the product is mainstream. Laggards are sceptical for an extended period of time but, eventually, adopt out of necessity, fearful of being called Luddites. These creatures of habit are against change and preach traditionalism until this position becomes untenable.

METCALFE'S LAW: THE WONDER OF NETWORKS

Metcalfe's law states: the value of a telecommunications network is proportional to the square of the number of connected users of the system (n^2).

Robert Metcalfe defined a law of great importance in the modern world that speaks to the effect of having linkages between people and machines that form a web of connectivity. This web allows many users to add value to the communication stream and mine the same data. When a few users are in the network, it has simple effects that allow the joiners to send messaging back and forth. The simple telephone connection was one of these in times past when there was no data-handling component and analog audio transmitted the message. Networks became more complex, big data was stored, and more was possible, so the innovators created the data world that we know as the Internet. The analysis of data and secondary big data effects suddenly became apparent. Once this system became large enough, it actually began to generate benefits that no one could anticipate. Benefits of "self-regulated learning" became important.

THE INTERNET OF THINGS

The concept of the Internet of Things (IoT) is that products, animals, people, and objects will have unique identifiers and transmit data over networks. This is good news for product functionality and reliability. The Gartner.com IoT report of 2013 predicts that by 2020 there will be 26 billion connected devices and objects. The network effect of this trend will create a new world order as yet not understood.

ANTIFRAGILITY: SYSTEMS THAT OUTPERFORM THEIR INVENTORS

Antifragility will be enabled by this trend as more producers follow the example of aircraft engine manufacturers and install sensors and connectivity to products so that "product learning" will create resilience.

The satellite reporting data stream emitted by modern jet aircraft and their engines is an example of a network effect. As the pilots and aircrew monitor and control flight, aircraft systems report regularly to an earthbound station. Location of the aircraft is transmitted by Mode-S transponders to an automatic dependent surveillance-broadcast (ADS-B) system paired with a global positioning system (GPS) that provides plane-to-plane aircraft separation data. Pilots are provided with real-time weather from satellite transmission, and the network records all for analysis of the system. A failure to separate aircraft is recorded for quality assurance activity. This aviation GPS system will replace the land-based radar system as radar increasingly takes a secondary role. The data-handling system will develop unintended benefits.

The concept of anti-fragility is for inventors and CEOs as we move into the new era of product development. Using Metcalfe's Law, we conceive of systems that have learning ability that continuously improves the performance and safety of the product that we develop.

There are three possible types of product:

- *Rugged durable products* that are designed to withstand regular abuse and challenging conditions. The Caterpillar tractor has brutally strong components that rarely fail.

- *Fragile products* designed with limited strength and resistance to stress. The teacup must be carefully handled and washed.
- *Antifragile products* that learn from experience in the world of disorder to thereby become stronger, smarter, and more likely to survive. The air traffic control system is becoming an antifragile system because the heart of the system is a computing hub that will analyze system performance and improve. Robotic systems with sensors and automatic functions can improve by learning about the environment they live in. The self-driving car is such a system if it begins to analyze your regular path to work, the traffic laws of your city, or your customary inputs.

Antifragile: Things That Gain from Disorder (Taleb, 2012) was written by Professor Nassim Nicholas Taleb. Applications have just begun to appear as smartness is designed into equipment. In my view, an attempt should be made with the development of each new product to add a learning system that could enhance function—for example, a device with sensors such as video with object recognition software that could decide what kind of coaching to provide to users. The device might learn to recognize who is currently driving the system. The coaching would change as the user learns more about the device. Lighting and video parameters could be enhanced as the device encounters changes.

CHANGING REGULATORY STANDARDS AND THE LEAN COMPLIANCE REQUIREMENT

Regulations are a reality for all industries, none more than the medical and aviation industries. Start-up founders must get good advice early to begin the learning process. The growth of company value and revenue makes the risk of regulatory misstep very costly. The R word (recall) is the most dreaded word in industry because the cost associated is so enormous. The recall pulls masses of product back from the market, results in a pressured root-cause analysis, distracts teams from product sales, detracts from a winning attitude, and hits the bottom line. The follow-up must deal with the engineering, design, and production issues to scrub the company for the future. Failure to do an exemplary job could lead to sagging growth and even bankruptcy. The medical company may reduce the complexity of regulation by limiting development to class 1 or class 2 products.

Lean regulatory processes are designed to protect the company from excessive burden and very slow development. The skill and magic come from regulatory process that enables rapid product development and does not slow launch. The regulatory team must have funding that allows complete verification and validation in a time frame that is acceptable.

Lean compliance begins with a clear definition of the product goals. These should be kept simple and lean enough to allow a simple list of features that converts into a specification profile. The profile itself is crafted to allow complete testing of the list in verification and validation. Design of the product must be created with the clear idea of how each feature will be tested to comply with design control. Product life expectancy must be defined and tested. All players must be at the table to take a linear view of the design and its path forward to keep the specifications clear and testable.

Verification testing assures that the specifications defined at the outset of the product development process have been achieved. Did we do an excellent job of achieving our technical goals? Validation testing affirms that the correct product has been built to address the medical need defined at the outset of the project. Did we build an effective product?

The verification and validation needs to assure that the strengths of the product are demonstrated and unacceptable rates of failure are prevented. Nothing made by humans is perfect. Two-thirds of the nonrecurring costs of a typical aerospace new product are spent on verification and validation. If this activity is poorly organized product launch will either be delayed forever or carried out with an unacceptable rate of failure.

Complex software planning platforms such as PLEXUS can be used in large entities to optimize compliance program logic. An estimated 80 percent of product life cycle cost is locked in at the end of the preliminary design phase.

TRAINING THE CEO

The selection of the CEO in start-ups is usually informal and depends on available resources. The CEO is always moving into uncharted waters that are filled with challenges. The leader must define the mission clearly and develop a business plan that will move inexorably to victory.

The ACETECH Growth Strategy Program in British Columbia is designed to mentor budding CEOs with a group learning format.

Founded in 1991, ACETECH is a unique example of a nongovernmental collaboration for CEOs. Participants are taught to create smart goals for the new corporation that will form the foundation of the company plans and behaviour. The CEO roundtable concept also encourages CEOs to meet regularly to bring sensitive topics to the table. Topics causing problems are not usually unique but have been experienced many times by our predecessors. This learning must be shared to prevent recurring errors by CEOs.

PHYSICIANS SKILL SETS	BUSINESS GRADUATE SKILL SET
Selected for intellect	Selected for intellect
Enthusiasm to achieve and contribute	Enthusiasm to achieve business growth
Advanced level education MD	Postgraduate education MBA
Deep knowledge base medicine with highly developed people caring skills	Advanced people-skills training and special business skills such as accounting and strategy creation.
Ethical focus on providing benefit to others	Ethical focus on providing benefit to the business and its growth.
Lifelong learning expectation	Lifelong learning expectation
Medical professional links	Extensive business networking

Fig. 18: Comparison between physician and business graduate skill sets.

Self-regulated learning for the CEO is key.

CEO TIME MANAGEMENT AND STRATEGY PRIORITIES

The CEO must use the "Business Model Canvas" to get to a business model describing how to operate the company as a product delivery system. How the company makes money will be a high priority when projecting possible growth curves. CEO time expenditure should fit with expressed goals and aspirations. It is a useful exercise to take a week to record time use and categorize it as family, business development, strategy thought, product innovation, and so forth to understand what these time allocations say about priorities. It is not uncommon to find that your time allocation doesn't match your expressed priority list.

Time is the executive's main asset in dealing with the needs of the company. Therefore, allocation and reallocation is the method of shifting the balance toward changing needs. The company generally has two streams of activity:

- activities that advance the business plan and reflect the expressed strategy
- activities that are unplanned and appear as problems not anticipated

The unplanned category should not be the predominant time consumer in the company. "Fire fighting" is a symptom of the failure to plan and suggests that a serious review is required. Personnel issues, product design deficiencies, quality control deficiencies, or other issues may require root cause analysis to prevent recurrence.

NEGOTIATING SKILLS

Negotiating is a skill that a CEO must master. Classic books such as *Getting to Yes* by Robert Fisher and William Ury teach a sophisticated approach to achieving a win-win outcome for a negotiation. Negotiating mistakes is costly. Every effort must be made to get training, which will also enhance negotiations with employees, other companies, finance providers, and service providers.

The best outcomes are achieved when you conceive and deliver a solution set for your adversary that solves the problem in a way that is innovative and adds unanticipated value to both parties. The goal is to leave the negotiation with a view to a future in which you may again collaborate with your negotiation partner to achieve ongoing business solutions. The ideal end point of the negotiation should improve the lot of both sides and produce the potential for long-lasting relationships.

Hardball negotiations may be unavoidable if the other side has people, attitudes, or needs that are difficult. Tricks such as eleventh-hour demands or sudden loss of momentum may occur. Should this happen, your plan to finesse the game by crafting creative solutions may be derailed. Take care to step back and request a time out to consider a response to this breach of trust. Resume negotiations with a plan that avoids emotion and personality but focuses on issues. If the demands are modest, consider accepting the change but do so as an equal. Readiness to walk away from hardball situations is a strong position and may be your "Plan B."

THE CONCEPT OF DISRUPTIVE INNOVATION

Clayton Christensen, professor at Harvard Business School, created the term *disruptive innovation*, which describes the effect of new ideas on the traditional methods of performing tasks and solving problems. Disruptive ideas change the competitive landscape.

The surgical example of a disruptive innovation would be laparoscopic surgery where 90 percent of a modern surgeon's work schedule was converted to video-mediated operations that were unexpectedly introduced.

The GlideScope was also disruptive in anaesthesia because it changed the American Society of Anesthesiologists (ASA) difficult airway management algorithm after consensus that video laryngoscopy was now an essential part of modern airway management.

The Harvard Business School group has many authors who have contributed to innovation knowledge. Innovation in modern business thinking has grown as companies wrestle with trying to keep growth alive. Copiers, or thieves, around the world make product life cycles shorter and shorter. Paradoxically, a true disruption needs time to create changes in behaviour. During new market creation, potential copiers usually sleep. Totally new products, by definition, have no market, so the start-up company needs to create change momentum.

The data storage paradigm is an example of disruptive innovation. Storage began in the previous century as a desk drawer and a file cabinet. Then came computer card storage, large data servers based on collections of tape storage, floppy discs such as the Winchester drive, minidiscs, solid-state storage such as the pervasive thumb drive, and now cloud-based storage such as Apple's I Cloud. Cloud-based storage relies on massive data centers requiring megawatts of power in server farms, which themselves are begging for disintermediation with yet another generation of data storage disruption. The product life cycle here is short, so profit must be taken early.

HR: CALIPER INTERVIEWS THAT GET PERSONAL

The right people in the right seats, doing the right thing, for the right reason is a way of emphasizing the huge importance of hiring excellence. Take advantage of trained HR professionals to vet potential employees and assure that the skill set matches the needs of the job. Testing methods for personnel assessment, such as the

Caliper test (calibercorp.com), measure personality traits and match them with unique corporate culture characteristics. Testing looks at a variety of metrics, such as aggressiveness, problem solving, skepticism, communicative style, assertiveness, impatience, and sense of urgency. Investigate to find the product that suits your needs. Verathon's experience with Caliper was interesting, effective, and accurate in my experience.

CORPORATE CULTURE

Tasks required of management include creating a corporate culture that advances the business model. Good corporate culture is a meritocracy free of nepotism and arcane features. The people you need to employ to develop and sell your ideas must be treated with fairness and rewarded with suitable income and family-friendly practices. Good work must be overtly recognized; poor performance should be managed in a way that gets it to acceptable levels. The trial employment period is your opportunity to find out quickly how well the employee fits the culture and job. Failure to achieve these levels promptly means the employee is a poor fit for the job. These individuals should be trained further or allowed to go to another enterprise where they will be effective. Management failure to deal fairly with employees who are underperforming places a burden on fellow workers and makes the workplace a conflict zone. The goal is to have well-managed employees who come happily to work and return to their families with energy and pride.

There is a need to achieve cultural fit with new employees. This can only be done when the organization teaches a culture that is accepted and provides a harmonious workplace, where people are able to verbalize the cultural tenets. Corporate culture must insist on mutually respectful conduct, no discrimination for the usual list of differences, adoption of company goals and strategies, ability to learn, and a desire to work toward company goals. Free thinking and debate are valuable assets, but they should eventually be set aside once the company has made a decision. Employees must then move forward aligned with company direction.

Management should take every opportunity to teach a set of goals and respond positively to the issues experienced by employees. As the company grows, a complaint hotline should be established to HR, which must find enlightened solutions to issues. Education and wellness programs are a vital part of ensuring alert, healthy, and engaged employees who will produce the highest quality product.

Culture is determined by the fundamental goals of the company. Such goals could be:

- growth targets with steady increases in profitability
- promoting a healthy happy workforce.
- providing a living wage.
- providing a safe workplace that does not permit any form of discrimination.
- making employees enthusiastic learners and funding learning opportunities.

While these may seem like "nice to have" goals, in fact, they are essential. Contented employees will work hard to defend an honourable company. The most profitable companies also have the finest people policies. I have worked for a large multinational where culture was reinforced by annual computerized retraining on major ethical topics. Real monitoring and action follows this annual training to assure that employees live up to the company's cultural norms. Good culture is teachable and builds a strong community.

Younger employees—millennials and Gen X, Y, and Z—have a new set of attitudes and priorities. Millennials will be the new wealth builders and are now on the move. Millennials are highly connected by Twitter, web-based e-mail, blogs, and other social media, and they are attracted to companies that eschew corporate social responsibility (CSR) and community. Older managers may miss a whole level of communication and complexity by being unaware of these connections. These communications may have more impact on the company image than, for example, paid advertising, which is usually carefully managed to control image. Workers will test the veracity of statements and assumptions in real time and make this known. The only defense against this testing is to have a clearly defined corporate culture that has inspiring goals. Management promotes culture by example and supports it by teaching and enforcing.

KOLS: IDENTIFYING AND ENGAGING THE TOP-TEN LEADERS.

The top-ten people in your customer base must be contacted and exposed to your product value equation and its potential early in development. This group will be at once very approachable, very smart, and very direct in giving feedback. Members of the top-ten group are usually distinguished from the majority by their need to be promoters of progress and disintermediation. The word *maven* describes these opinion leaders, who need to know every detail of their specialty and need to be the agents of change.

A certain amount of aggressiveness is needed to chase down and get attention from a busy academic physician, who, typically, has clinical obligations, teaching schedules, publishing needs, and administrative work. With the GlideScope development, I found that the nursing and office gatekeepers are likely to help when the caller is an MD. I would often ask where the individual was and then call the OR or clinic to make contact. I rarely failed to speak to even the loftiest individual for a few minutes. These individuals are usually very alert and can quickly decide whether or not they wish to be involved with your mission. Corporate leaders will usually be accessible to an MD as well, because the gatekeepers don't know if the call is from a golf partner, a personal physician, or a business associate. When talking to a senior business leader, expect a rapid decision on the relevance of your call to the business. If there is any interest, you will immediately be passed to a senior deputy at the VP level who will be directed to report back on the opportunity. The senior VP will usually do a high-level review of your topic and report back to the superior.

Never begin at the middle or the bottom of an organization because an enormous amount of luck and work will be required to power your idea up to the decision maker level. It will likely not happen. Therefore, you always start at the top.

Note: The early development of Saturn Biomedical was greatly influenced by two anaesthesia experts: Dr. John Doyle and Dr. Richard Cooper from the University of Toronto and Toronto Hospital. The initial contact with these leaders was brief but meaningful. They were interested in our goals and patient to assist with our uncertain start. The majority of individuals are happily living their lives and are not great advocates of change but, rather, tend to use and be satisfied with established, time-honoured approaches. This majority will not help you very much or at all.

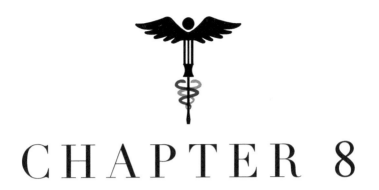

CHAPTER 8

COMPANY REQUIREMENTS FOR EXCELLENCE IN BUSINESS PROCESSES

The creation of Saturn Biomedical and thence Verathon Medical Canada forced me onto a learning path that relied heavily on the ACETECH Vancouver area CEO's group. Verne Harnish is a favourite speaker and thought leader for this group. The educational efforts of ACETECH include regular CEO lectures, CEO roundtable group coaching, and an annual meeting in Whistler that features international speakers and workshops. My education from this group included extensive methodology for building a positive corporate culture. Acetech teaches how to create a working, scalable business model that can form the basis for a growth strategy.

ROCKEFELLER HABITS MODERNIZED

Mastering the Rockefeller Habits: What You Must Do to Increase the Value of Your Growing Firm by Verne Harnish describes how to establish a communication rhythm that will configure a company for rapid growth. The rhythm of business is part of the culture of a business and can be deliberately planned and established. The Rockefeller habits rhythm is patterned after the behaviour of ascetic Baptist John D. Rockefeller Jr. and his three sons. These leaders developed consistent behaviour patterns. They walked to the office each morning together and by so doing integrated the activities of a far-flung business empire. Their diverse holdings in key industries benefitted from the daily brief collaboration, which, in effect, provided a consultation and transfer of facts in a day when personal contact was the primary means of communication, supplemented by letters and memos.

This behaviour has been replicated by many tech businesses in the form of:

1. Daily Stand-up Meeting

The stand-up meeting brings together the leadership team for 15 minutes. The question, why are we paying you today? is answered. The answer describes what you plan for your contribution and how it might fit with the established goals and today's needs. These meetings can be carried out at multiple levels to effect alignment with the larger goals articulated by management. The stand-up format is important because these meetings must not drag on or solve problems; they are designed to provide day-to-day focus on the business now.

2. Weekly Meetings

At these meetings, problems are discussed in depth and solved. Regular encounters make it easy for the leader to repeat the mission focus and detect low levels of achievement. In the end, a rather amorphous group can become a serious force that is highly integrated and effective by establishing rhythm.

Rhythm and organization must originate and be led from the top. Discipline is required to assure that the rhythm persists. The effect of this kind of team discipline is that communication is direct, in the open, measurable by peers, and has no need of other sublevels of communication to accomplish tasks. Politics must be minimized by adherence to an open meritocracy. The enterprise has little excess resources, as a rule, and therefore only gets a few chances to build the next great product or process. While the C-level leaders must have an intimate appreciation of how the product under development perfectly fills the needs of the customer and ensure that it is produced, any incursions into the tasks of the juniors is demotivating and provokes the question, if you do my work why do you pay me? The properly selected employee, given freedom to find flexible solutions to daily problems, will usually give much more than expected and need not be micro-managed.

3. Regular Reporting to Your Leader

The management structure should rely on a simple organization chart with no dotted lines of confusion. Subordinates must request a regular meeting to get approval for their plans. They must meet their superior with an agenda and present the status quo of their part of the business, their plan to execute the mission, and an account of their department's budget. Failure to present a plan worthy of approval would mean a return meeting to get organized. The bottom line is that you must manage your unit and not rely on direction from above. Goals, pointers, comments, and approval are all you get. The senior manager must have the discipline to wait for the report to present uncontested plans.

The cultural rhythm must also limit duplication of effort and *muda* (Japanese for "futility") resulting from micro-management from the top. If senior leaders spend time to guide, correct, or motivate certain employees, they must ask if such employees are suited to their job. According to my mentor, Gerald McMorrow, the ex-CEO of Verathon Medical, a company with $200 million in annual revenue, the number of direct reports a manager can handle is limited to six or seven. This was true at Verathon Canada, where a great culture rhythm was established.

THE METRONOME EFFECT: MANAGEMENT RHYTHMS THAT CREATE AND SUSTAIN ALIGNMENT

The metronome effect is a concept developed by Shannon Berne Susko and described in her book *The Metronome Effect: The Journey to Predictable Profit* (Susko, 2014). The metronome keeps musicians on a regular beat that creates a rhythm similar to that which occurs in a company when the executive team is culturally aligned and making its benchmark goals. It's an extension of the Rockefeller habits and rhythm. Susko, CEO of Paradata Systems before becoming CEO of Subserveo, the Internet payment service, believes that you need to consciously recognize a "personal *why*." This is the analytical, emotional answer for why you come to work each day. What is driving you? What is your goal?

- Some wish to create a company to solve a large problem, such as Elizabeth Holmes, CEO of Theranos, a medical company with an income of US$9 billion. Holmes is driven to disintermediate the hospital and private laboratory world with a disruptive innovation using microfluidics and microchemistry to automatically do blood analysis with a single drop of blood.

- Some wish to make a life-changing amount of money to enable the freedom to be with their family for a critical growth period.

- Some wish to make a contribution to the medical world to enhance their self-esteem and make them feel worthy.

- Some wish to build a great company and exercise creative management genius, an approach known as builder psychology. This will usually be associated with extraordinary wealth earned as growth occurs.

- Some labour for the love of business. Warren Buffett appears to be a person of this type. Business is addictive when it is done well. The delight of success is a powerful driver.

THE MENTOR EFFECT

Modern business thinking incorporates mentoring as a necessity, even at the highest levels of the organization. There is a need for education at all levels. CEOs need a strong mentor as much as the midlevel executive or junior employee because their lifelong learning concept must be entrenched. There is a need for timely and regular counsel from those who are peers.

The obvious issue is how to reach out to choose a suitable mentor and arrange the relationship to the benefit of the person being mentored. CEOs' skill and intelligence are all that protect them. CEOs have the final authority to decide which policies will be recommended to the board of directors, and the mentor at this point is not a factor. Mentoring is best carried out by the most skilled and clever person available because CEOs have the fate of all of the employees in their hands. In a perfect world a mentor will identify with the mission and contribute selflessly.

FINANCING A SUCCESSFUL ENTERPRISE

The start-up company is a temporary construct with the mission of defining the first product and creating the first straw man business model, which defines how to get money with the product. Bootstrapping describes a method of growing a start-up for an extended period of time using founder resources. The definition implies little or no external input, similar to pulling yourself up by your own bootstraps. The advantages of bootstrapping are many. Patience and sweat equity are needed to power product customization for the first customers. This focus allows you to learn to become intimate with the needs of the customers and learn how each benefit of your product is valued.

1. Patience to get proof of your business model rewards founders with higher equity.
2. The founders learn to get the business model right.
3. The founders are in total control when they need to be.

The general sequence of financing begins with "love money" provided by friends and family to give the founders the chance to start the business. The funds contributed generally allow you to produce a series of prototypes of product and a first business model.

Failure of start-up companies is common, so bootstrapping is fraught with risk of impact on the social base of the inventors.

The next level investment is provided by angel investors, who take positions in start-up companies in the hope of having a few successes that yield a tenfold return on invested capital. These investors are often led by an experienced investor who has a significant, positive record of success with previous ventures. The classic time required for actualization of a company is in the range of ten years, so ideally, the investor group must have a longer time horizon and an appetite for risk. The goal of early investors should be to think in terms of making successive early tranches of contribution to keep the company on a path with continued momentum. This kind of high-risk investment must be guided by a clear vision of the successive target goals of the management, which will serve as triggers for subsequent advances. Angel investors like to have a clear idea of the exit strategy envisioned by the company but must realize that most success stories require ten or more years. Having said this, most angels have preference for extracting most of their invested capital early with the option of leaving equity in place to participate in the growth phase when most value is created.

STAGES OF INVESTMENT

1. Self-financing to begin:

- Bootstrap as far as you can: owner has 100 percent.
- Friends and family provide love money; owner has 90 percent.

2. Seed money: owner sells 10 to 15 percent and retains 80 percent.

- $1 to $2 million: take as little as possible.
- This money sets you up for venture rounds and introduces venture groups.

3. Venture rounds to power growth:

- Round A to power growth may be 20 percent.
- Round B follow-through is based on benchmarks at 12 percent.

4. Company powers its own growth and has organic growth:

- The company can borrow money for growth, or
- The company can do a version of customer-financed growth in which specialty product is developed with the customer, IP rights staying with the company. With this mode, loyalty is due to the contract customer, but you can fund product and business model development with customer money.

New money may be a saviour or an elixir of death, depending on the conditions required by the financial contributor. The new management team may need money so acutely that any source may seem to be acceptable, especially if it comes from a large entity. Clayton Christensen and Michael Raynor, in their book *The Innovator's Solution* (Christensen and Raynor, 2013), have a useful chapter on good and bad money.

The complex process of going to capital providers requires that the company objectives be well conceived and articulated. The business model to move to commercialization must be credible and detailed with use of a classic Gantt chart to allow the investors to understand the steps involved. This secondary investor group must be approached with the understanding that:

- The start-up is a temporary construct with the mission of defining a product and a business model. At this point, a classic business plan is conjecture.
- It is essential that the founders retain a meaningful interest.
- Follow-through financings can be accomplished without the need to do a down round or reduced share value offering by continuing to add significant value so that the investor group remains comfortable with the progress of the enterprise.
- Ideally, the investor group will buy into the risk points and step up with more money during challenging times without punishing the team.

GOOD MONEY

1. According to Christensen and Raynor, good money is "patient for growth but impatient for profitability." This notion recognizes that the only way to get the product right is to perfect it for customers so they will pay a price with a good margin. Profit earned is tangible evidence that early customer targeting is successful and the team is operating with a model built to satisfy at least one real customer.

2. Good money is provided in timely fashion triggered by achieving planned benchmarks.

3. Good money may enable a successful acquisition when the new company's contribution falls clearly in the strategic path of a larger company. The problem faced by the larger company is that truly disruptive ideas usually reside outside the walls of the company in what Henry Chesbrough calls "the sea of ideas" in the open innovation model.

4. Good money is not linked to outdated thinking or advice.

5. Good money is linked to understanding the innovation and how it may be disruptive.

BAD MONEY

1. Bad money is impatient for simultaneous growth and profitability, which is unrealistic when the product is truly disruptive and must take time to create a market.

2. Bad money is coupled with bad guidance.

3. Bad money may be from corporate sources that, by application of their own business model, force the configuration of the new company and its product away from being disruptive.

4. Bad money may wish to "pump and dump" the new company by making an early profitable exit. The fast money team can severely damage the young company by causing a momentum stall.

5. Bad money may have insufficient depth to continue to support the new disruptive innovation to a point where others can take over.

6. Bad money can establish control and, in effect, park the technology.

In summation, the character of the funding source is critical to the long-term outcome. Goodwill and trust are required to allow the core team time to experiment with the business model and product.

The sources of venture capital need to understand how the idea or invention will solve a problem with a significant market size. The product should enable the establishment of a company with a strong patent base that will lead to growth in sales, margin, and profit. This will enable a profitable exit for capital, which will then be re-tasked for other worthy projects. When a business has solid growth, most capital will stay in place to participate in value growth.

It is important for the start-up company to keep the company coffers filled with enough cash that the burn rate will extend for one or more years without replenishment. Management must be able, at all times, to know and control the burn rate. The most common technique for this is to limit credit card use and have the CEO personally sign all cheques. This is possible for a very long time during company growth.

When more capital is required by the business model, it is best acquired before it is needed. Should management become desperate, there is the possibility of a down round of financing. This will be irritating for early investors because the value of their initial investment will be reduced and the founders will suffer equity punishment. Management must create a tempo of achievement of hard targets that will reassure early investors and encourage subsequent contributions to complete the company mission.

At times, it is possible to get investment from a large company that is manoeuvring to be in an advantageous position if the product or drug is successful. The general posture of large entities is to purchase projects after the product has been validated in the marketplace to the extent that delivery of a demonstrated ROI can be predicted at the time of purchase. Large entities such as Johnson & Johnson need to see a substantial revenue stream from the product and business model before they would consider acquisition. Occasionally the investment may be necessary to block a competitor or build on a vital strategic priority. The upstart that approaches these large players will almost always be disappointed. It is still probably worth doing a presentation if invited, even though it may just end up being an educational opportunity for the acquirer's research and development executives. Investors are very keen that the start-up company has intelligent leadership with high-quality mentoring. Then, should significant reverses occur in the course of business, a sharp and capable team will find a way to have a phoenix rise from the ashes and make another attempt at success. A quality management team will have significant depth with capable people in key positions such as finance, engineering, and operations.

A weak team is unattractive to acquirers because team rebuilding is time consuming, management intensive, and risky. Hidden misery that may reside in the poorly managed entity is potentially costly. Management that produces a great culture with successive quarters of growth or goal achievement is probably capable of staying out of trouble.

What Do We Learn about Financing?

1. Investors must realize that a start-up is a temporary construct with a mission to perfect product and find a suitable business model.
2. The quality and skill of the mentored leadership team will be critical to the survival of a start-up.
3. The CEO should sign all cheques and control credit cards to keep the burn rate at a level that the company can afford.
4. When seeking money, be prepared to give a single-sentence description of what you do better than anyone else.
5. Never run out of money; have one year's worth secured.
6. Never take more financing money than you need, but add a margin of safety.
7. Swimming with sharks is dangerous to your health. Always deal with high-quality investors and business partners.
8. Bootstrap your company as far as possible, using as much of your own resources as possible. Financial supporters will give a higher valuation when the early achievements have clearly defined the customer, potential market size, and the product.
9. Sweat equity is the best kind of equity for start-ups.
10. Consider the possibility of a customer-funded business model, like Airbnb, as a means to avoid financing dilution.
11. Consider the invention of a subscription revenue business model. Amazon can assist start-ups with subscription revenue sales. The subscription gives the service at a known cost and avoids a purchase decision.

NAMING AND BRANDING AS RESERVOIRS OF VALUE

The building of a product and company results in substantial value. Identification of the company with this value begins to confer brand equity. The development of a conscious brand image is important and constitutes one of the important executive functions that can extend the life of the company. Brand decisions can result in production of an image that becomes stronger with the addition of successive generations of products. Brand equity will add value to the company upon its sale.

The branding discussion around Verathon and Saturn Biomedical began when Saturn was sold to Diagnostic Ultrasound in 2006. The first discussions were mediated by a branding consultant in meetings focused on defining the type of people present in the newly amalgamated entity. The name Diagnostic Ultrasound did not encompass both the ultrasound products and the airway product GlideScope. A new name would need to be selected.

Verathon had a disciplined achiever culture in both companies. The united company was aiming to be a house of brands, wherein the product names were emphasized rather than the new company name. The Verathon name was subordinated to brand recognition of the Bladderscan and the GlideScope to allow the addition of new brands with brand power encapsulated in each product line. This idea seemed to work well for the period of growth of the two united brands. Sales were climbing rapidly for GlideScope and were climbing steadily for the more mature Bladderscan ultrasound. The name search became a long process of elimination that ended when we combined the concepts of *veritas* (seeking truth) with the idea of *marathon* (going the distance) into Verathon. This portmanteau strategy was cheerfully adopted.

THE POWER OF BRAND ARCHETYPES

The description of psychological archetype behaviour was initiated by Karl Jung, who recognized that 12 behaviours are constant models recognized and understood through the ages. The archetypes have been the basis for stories, myths, and sagas used to portray generic ideals. These behaviour patterns carry with them emotive power that can be harnessed by branding. The company capitalizes on the idea of the brand by consciously choosing and adhering to the features of the archetype. In *The Hero and the Outlaw: Building Extraordinary Brands through the Power of Archetypes* (2001), authors Margaret Mark and Carol Pearson discuss the use of classical archetypes to create powerful brands.

According to Mark and Pearson, the 12 master brand archetypes are:

1. innocent: utopian and free;
2. sage: the truth will set you free;
3. explorer: don't fence me in;
4. ruler: authoritarian;
5. creator: creates enduring value;
6. caregiver: cares for others;
7. magician: dreams large;
8. hero: takes action to help and rescue others;
9. outlaw: anger; rules are to be broken;
10. lover: builds intimacy and experience;
11. jester: creates fun and enjoyment;
12. regular guy/gal: ordinary

Famous brand ideas incorporated into well-known companies include the magician brand of Disney, which creates wonder and excitement from use of the imagination. The mentor brands of Oprah and Martha Stewart promise to give life guidance and mothering while conveying trust. The outlaw brands that promise to break the rules with excitement and adventure are embodied in Harley-Davidson and Apple. The jester brands of Pepsi and Coors promise fun and enjoyment while being light-hearted.

BRANDING VERATHON MEDICAL AND PRODUCTS

The next decision was to select a brand archetype we could identify with. This process was achieved by reference to our two unique products adding much clinical value to the medical profession and their patients. This led to discussion of whether we should be a hero brand or a caregiver brand. We chose the hero brand because the contribution of the products was preventing airway disasters with GlideScope and preventing urinary obstruction and urinary tract infections with the Bladderscan.

Armed with our new hero brand, a new innovation was acquired, the HeartScape 80-lead EKG. This product was designed to enable emergency caregivers to diagnose myocardial infarcts by applying the system. A computerized data-handling component produced a powerful graphic presentation of ischemia on a color monitor that could diagnose 25 percent more ST-segment elevation myocardial infarction (STEMI) patterns, especially in the posterior zones of the heart. This allowed for timely angioplasty and stenting to save heart muscle in these heart-attack victims.

The hero brand would match this product very well because a full 25 percent of patients were likely to be diagnosed more rapidly.

The company would adopt a heroic posture and would save many lives in the future should this work be successful. The program was delayed because of execution issues. The branding effort, however, was well conceived and carried forward. The development of the brand concept relied heavily on the work of Mark and Pearson.

Brand is important because customers want to find a reliable, delightful brand to add value to their life and then move on without repeatedly examining this need. Brands are more powerful than ever in a cluttered marketplace where differentiators are badly needed.

PRODUCT NAMING STRATEGY

An abundance of literature and learning materials are associated with legions of consultants employed to create a value-adding name. Naming brings up questions that bear on the market, the business model, and a host of other ideas.

Bladderscan has become a very successful descriptive name for the clinical application as well as the product.

The GlideScope is an evocative name suggesting that the video product will lead you to a successful target. The aviation-based name guides aircraft to a successful landing while the medical device guides the anaesthesiologist to a successful intubation of the airway. Appropriation strategy conveys the benefit of another recognizable benefit from a different field. The GlideScope name was selected over the common medical strategy of naming the product after the inventor to secure that person's place in history.

Names and brands confer the following benefits when selected successfully.

1. They strategically distinguish a unique position in the market.
2. They offer trademark and legal benefits.
3. They, ideally, appeal to the target audience in some clever way.
4. They are easy to say and remember.
5. They carry meaning and may become an overriding name like Xerox, Kleenex, and Pampers.
6. They allow platform-naming opportunities when new product is introduced.

EXIT STRATEGY CONSIDERATIONS

The exit planning should begin when you do your first real task for the company. Tell yourself that your company is being built to sell. Years later you will have done a great many tasks to make the company attractive for your buyer. Sell your company when the time is right from a company-value point of view, along with other considerations such as shareholders wishes. Legal advisors should be well prepared because of your foresight.

Become proactive and seek a buyer who would benefit by adding your company to the blend of products or services that buyer now provides. The acquirer's sales channel should accommodate the new products without large investment, and the competencies should be approximately correct. The other company will often be visible to you in your space. Find a champion in the company who sees the value of acquisition. As with any negotiation, you must know the other company's position accurately so that you can enable an excellent plan for it. Planning will lead to greater value and higher price. The strategy to sell should include reaching out to all companies operating in the space. Those who would benefit competitively from purchase may not be aware of the potential sale. Ideally, create a bidding situation that will generate urgency and have a favourable effect on the final sale price.

The company value includes the business intellectual property, the business model, the earning stream and the goodwill with customers and suppliers. These values must be backed up with a solid legal foundation that includes important NDA files, employment agreements, consulting agreements, and shareholder agreements that describe the exchanges for services and payments, all signed at the time of the agreements. Should these be deficient, some contractor or employee could hold your sale for ransom at the very last minute and extract onerous payment with some kind of challenge. In short, do your homework from the beginning of your adventure.

The larger the acquiring company is, the more able it will be to pay, but such a company will want a detailed record of sales and market success. The larger company needs unrelenting growth without risk. Ideally, the acquirer will see a couple of years of momentum in the entity as well as a platform for growth that can be guided toward improvement in the return on invested equity. The acquired company should be able to earn enough to pay a good cash return annually while retaining enough cash for the team to develop the platform potential.

The "mergers suck and acquisitions rock" adage comes from the notion that an acquired company with intact management and previous history of momentum will likely continue to achieve in a similar way, unless the management is destabilized. Merging cultures is a high-risk activity that can be avoided by allowing the existing management team to continue doing the magic work that made them desirable in the beginning. Destabilization can be caused by the acquirer or by the seller of the acquired company if, as Warren Buffet says, the seller "loves money more than the company."

Buffet allegedly uses an assessment of the passion of the acquired management team for the mission of the company as a metric when assessing acquisitions. When merging occurs between two business cultures, the risk of destroying value and losing the acquired property value is high. A merged entity is difficult to track and manage for determination of ROI increase.

The practice of buying great companies with great management and allowing them to continue to prosper without interference is the preferred route. This requires that the acquirer understands the business model and tracks performance while allowing the value creation process to continue. There are many possible ways of creating post-acquisition value increase, including sale of product lines and disassembly of the company, but the key is to recognize the essence of the business value creation model and assure that management capability can be retained while change is contemplated.

> *It's far better to buy a wonderful company at a fair*
> *price than a fair company at a wonderful price.*
> —Warren Buffet, letter to shareholders, 1989

The sale of Compilr, a Canadian software company that teaches coding, to Lynda.com in 2014 was aided by finding a second bidder. Through the existence of this second bid, the resulting negotiations moved the price in a positive direction to a reported $20 million. The 26-year-old CEO and founder expressed the view that he had spent too little time investigating Lynda.com and he regretted this oversight. The more you know about the adversary and its problems, the more likely you will be to assess the situation and provide deeper benefits to it to get the optimal price.

Price is not the only item to be traded upon. Variables can include the timing of payments, the expected tenure of the senior management, the likelihood that the newly purchased company will be physically moved, and the extent to which the merging of assets is possible.

Should both parties believe that the match will have a strong ROI for the acquirer, fair pay will be more likely. Usually, you will be dealing with an acquisition team that has previous experience to draw on, so try to find out what this previous experience is.

Use experienced legal advice that can appear at the table as your resource. Do not agree to surrender anything of significance at the early meetings. Rather, regard these as fact-gathering exercises. You need to understand, from the acquirer's viewpoint, how valuable the merged or acquired asset will be. If you ask repeatedly, there is a good chance that you will learn enough about the acquirer's business model to see its method of value creation. Education via books such as *Getting to Yes* by Roger Fischer and William Ury will allow you to design a creative solution in consultation with your legal team. Shift negotiation away from personality toward substantial facts, searching for positive value for both parties to agree upon. The needs of the parties to a negotiation are never symmetrical. One party may need timing advantages, one party may have a substantial tax problem, another party may need a small down payment, and so on.

The perfect negotiation could produce a final agreement that is non-adversarial and gives each party what they actually need.

The enemy of this type of outcome is lack of trust between parties. The more enlightened negotiator may need to teach the attitudes involved in getting to a mutual agreement that has major benefits for each side. The idea that there will be a winner and a loser is the worst outcome because you will fail to create trust. The more you know about yourself, the more experience you employ (including mentoring, coaching, expert assistance) and the more you know about the other side (character and business detail), the more likely you will be to make a deal.

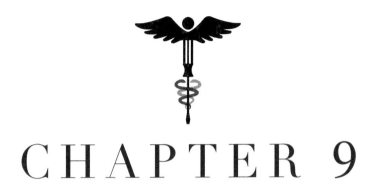

CHAPTER 9

SALES: THE FINAL COMMON PATHWAY

SALES STRATEGY

Selection of your sales leadership DNA is a profound decision and will determine your fate. Err here and you will be set back seriously or fail. The leader must craft your sales system and hire the "starving lions" sales team DNA, the most important single act for getting good results. The leadership must get the incentive structure in place for sales with targets based on profitability and individual performance. The question is how much each person contributes to profitability. Low achievers should be replaced promptly to get the right mindset in place.

A strong product makes superior sales performance easier to achieve. Document how effectively sales get in front of qualified customers with the value proposition. The classic sales funnel is created by good people presenting a great product to qualified customers able to pay the price for the product. Repeat sales add ease to the selling process by avoiding the need to educate new customer candidates. Sales team members must be chosen to favour those who know how to close with a sense of urgency and develop a lasting relationship with the customer.

ONLINE SALES: ZAPPOS' FIVE TENETS

Tony Hsieh of Zappos wrote an exceptional book, titled *Delivering Happiness: A Path to Profits, Passion, and Purpose* (Hsieh, 2010), on treating customers like royalty. I went to visit the Las Vegas call center to discover how this is done and was impressed by the buy-in of the staff as they discussed their performance targets and freedom to creatively serve the customer. I would strongly recommend a tour of this bastion of customer satisfaction.

Zappos' performance culture is a disciplined center of high energy and fun for workers who are charged with "delighting" online customers and then ringing the sales bell to create an air of excitement among the team.

Seventy-five percent of Zappos orders come from return customers. How does Zappos achieve this, and how can your company achieve the same stellar results?

1. Treat customers as individuals and have a solid scalable customer relationship management (CRM) system to keep track.

2. Empower employees to be creative when solving customer problems.

3. Do the unexpected to delight the customer and socialize this within the company to make it culture.

4. Reward repeat customers with exceptional kindness.

5. Never argue about returns. Plan for them and be quick with service.

6. Define what lightning-fast response means in responding to questions and customer issues. E-mails from customers are like fire alarms.

SATISFY ONE CUSTOMER PERFECTLY AND BECOME A CREATIVE LONG-TERM PARTNER WITH THAT CUSTOMER

Peter Drucker is core reading for those wishing to understand business model development. Drucker coined the term "knowledge worker" to describe someone who creates, understands, stores, teaches, and utilizes knowledge. Peter Drucker, once CEO of General Motors, produced legendary growth and taught a generation of business leaders the core values of management. Peter Drucker teaches that "the goal of business is to create and keep a customer."

The modern world is often portrayed as a place where brand doesn't matter and customer loyalty isn't as important as it once was. There is some truth to this notion, but there is another reality about the customer thought process. The customer is assaulted with information about products, processes, and brands in a continuous stream of loudly asserted images and ideas. The sheer volume of information makes it impossible to study and assess so the customer is left with an impossible task. The customer wants to make a decision once and tends to settle on a brand once chosen.

SALES AND MARKETING

1. Hire hunter DNA, no pussy cats; we want starving lions.
2. Successful sales people tap on their customers as many as eight times to connect.
3. Focus totally on the needs of this customer, such that you know what the customer needs better than the customer does. To do this you must learn and understand your customer's business completely.
4. The highest achievement is to have two-way communication established. Sales staff must be scripted educators of the customer while, at the same time, developing a continuous flow of knowledge about the customer's needs back to the company. Sales can identify mavens and educators who will distribute the company message.
5. Can you offer the best solution, the timely solution, when it is needed? If not, learn how.
6. Build lasting relationships with customers to become creative partners.
7. Delight your customer and use culture to incorporate and celebrate this.

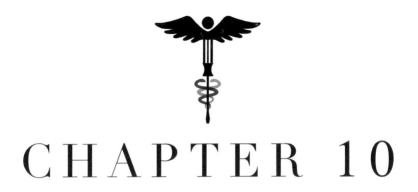

CHAPTER 10

HIRING "THE ARMY OF THE WILLING"

The quality of your key people will determine
how you will execute on strategy.
The army of the willing: find people who
want to be involved in your quest.
No sceptics and no toxic people, please.

Those with inherent enthusiasm will join projects they believe have great potential to benefit humanity, their bank account, or their need to contribute. When you are looking for support, money, excellent employees, or partners, you must wait and select those who fit the profile of the army of the willing. The "heart" of these people will drive them to work long and hard to create the great corporate culture you need. The corporate culture piece is vital to sustain a business life devoid of unnecessary grief and stress.

The start-up has a special problem with hiring because there is no reserve money or energy. A bad hire can lead to failure of the enterprise. It's better to not hire than to act quickly and hire someone with no "heart." If you even think about the question of firing, you should regard this as a flag and, after due thought, carry out the act.

Firing is difficult and should be done early when an employee

1. doesn't share the team vision;
2. is a poor performer not responding to coaching;
3. requires too much management;
4. causes political issues and disharmony;
5. is a sceptical individual seeding discontent.

The members of a team may be shocked by a firing, but if the cause is just, they appreciate the reasons and are reassured. Toxic people must exit. When people leave, you are doing them and your company a service. People who do not contribute rely on the hard work of fellow team members; the workload falls on the hard workers.

Hire:

- people with "heart"
- people with character who finish tasks with determination
- people who have "the right attitude and cultural team fit first and for skills and experience second" (Paul Geyer).
- people who are smarter than you will make you look good.

- people who come highly recommended by their previous manager.
- people whose references check out.

Nepotism is your enemy because you are unlikely to get the best person for the job.

TOPGRADING YOUR WAY TO SUCCESS IN HIRING

A good practice for hiring uses the teachings of Dr. Brad Smart to improve hiring success. The number-one determinant of success in the growth of companies is the number of high performers who are recruited. In his book *Topgrading 201: How to Avoid Costly Mis-Hires,* Brad Smart gives proven strategies for improving the hiring process. His basic text is *Topgrading* (Smart, 2012). Take the Topgrading training program.

TOPGRADING CAREER HISTORY FORM

The chronological Topgrading interview technique is recommended. How the candidate developed over time is the question. By using the Topgrading Career History form rather than relying on CV information, you will identify the candidates most likely to pass the interview. The history looks at each full-time job to find salaries, boss ratings, likes and dislikes in jobs, and the real reason for leaving employers. The truth serum inherent in the application of this document is that the assertions will be tested.

THE TOPGRADING INTERVIEW

The first interview in the Topgrading strategy is a basic competency interview and lasts one hour. The second interview is the custom chronological interview, conducted with reference to the Topgrading interview guide. Senior-level job interviews are conducted by two interviewers. Starting with each job in sequence, the candidate is asked to discuss accomplishments, failures and mistakes, appraisals by bosses, key decisions, and relationships.

Comprehensive reference checks are essential to confirm what is learned from the interview process. Do not rely on the candidate's hand-picked references. Ask the candidate to arrange an interview for you with the previous boss to confirm the interview findings directly. The cost of a mis-hire could easily exceed the annual salary of the individual, and the long-lasting embedded effects may be subtle.

CONCLUSION

SIGNIFICANT INVENTION CHANGES YOUR LIFE AND THE WORLD FOREVER

The GlideScope device was successful in powering Saturn Bio-medical Systems and then Verathon Medical because it was clinically excellent, solving the unmet need around difficult airway management. The companies had determined medical and business leadership and were adequately financed. Key physicians alerted the airway community that this new device was, like the LMA, a major contribution to patient safety.

The great inventors in this book made a conscious decision to become creative and build a new world. The drive to innovate and invent changed their lives. Their infectious enthusiasm changed those around them and engaged them in a journey. The description by Archie Brain of "Life after the LMA Invention" shows that a complete life change occurred driven by the momentum of an idea.

- The idea becomes more important than the inventor. This tests the ability of the inventor to learn to adapt to a rapidly changing life.
- Business life is supercharged, so inventors must become lifelong learning machines, driven to succeed.
- The lives of the great inventors demonstrate that choosing cofounders is a critical determinant of a venture's success and must be done with great care.

- The medical inventors discussed in this book energized people because everyone seeks meaning in life, and a medical cause is like no other. They mastered the skills of communication, innovation, and invention to get more satisfaction from life.

- Medical schools need to offer medical innovation course material. The new physician must be sparked to venture into the worlds of inventiveness and organizational management in an effective way.

- The spirit of inventive people creates a drive to leave a legacy based on a passionate contribution to science, affairs of state, and the science of minimizing pain and suffering. The desire to leave their mark was very strong.

- Inventors demonstrate that "a journey of a thousand miles can begin with a single step."

- Hire people who are smarter than you to embrace the passion that you bring to the mission. These people will determine the future success of your company and will be your most important asset.

CLOSING THOUGHTS

Physicians have an abundant urge to contribute to medical science. The guidelines to become innovators should be taught in modern medical schools. Physicians will be the focus of continuous change in the future. Physicians are pressed to keep their family life together while under a constant challenge from other influences and demands. Research shows that "burnout" is a significant mid-practice event that may become a catalyst for change.

Begin inventive life early because, over time, more and more focus can be placed on creative growth. Once the spirit of exploration takes hold, it becomes a prominent life force. The optimal time for inventiveness is when you begin to entertain the idea. The inventors discussed in this book teach that the excitement of being creative can result in contributions that produce far-reaching benefits for physicians and their patients. The invention path sparks a creative zeal that projects positive life energy to others. An early start enables greater contributions that can continue long after the inventive activity ceases as others build on the platform the inventor has created.

Inventiveness may develop later in professional life, when the pressing needs of a medical career become controlled and time is available for exploration and experimentation. Insights and unexpected events can propel you, as an inventor, in new directions. Importantly, when you begin a new knowledge journey, your life will change even if you do not have initial success with your ideas. Reward comes from the knowledge that you have done your best to live a life of change, taking opportunity to teach the young.

Encourage those with an idea to take that first step. The journey becomes a never-ending quest that takes you to places you would have never dreamed possible and introduces you to people you would not have otherwise met. Dr. Seuss said it all in *Oh, the Places You'll Go!* when he urged children to say yes to exploration. This applies to us all; create and chase your passion.

Exploration is critical for change. Ask only, "Where is my blue ocean at this time?"

The creative journey will flower into massive learning, reading, mentoring, teaching, and development.

BIBLIOGRAPHY

Abraham, Joe. 2011. *Entrepreneurial DNA: The Breakthrough Discovery That Aligns Your Business to Your Unique Strengths*. New York: McGraw Hill.

Brain, A. I. J. 1983. "The Laryngeal Mask Airway: A New Concept in Airway Management." *British Journal of Anaesthesia* 55 (8): 801–4.

Brain, A. I. J. 1985. "Three Cases of Difficult Intubation Overcome by the Laryngeal Mask Airway." *Journal of Anaesthesia* 40 (May): 353–55.

Brunton, Laurence, Bruce Chabner, and Bjorn Knollman. 2011. *Goodman and Gilman's Pharmacological Basis of Therapeutics*. New York: McGraw-Hill.

Canadian Consortium for Self-Regulated Learning, SRL Canada.

Chesbrough, Henry. 2003. *Open Innovation: The New Imperative for Creating and Profiting from Technology*. Boston: Harvard Business Review Press.

Christensen, Clayton M. 2011. *The Innovator's Dilemma: The Revolutionary Book That Will Change the Way You Do Business*. New York: Harper Business.

Christensen, Clayton M., and Michael E. Raynor. 2013. *The Innovator's Solution: Creating and Sustaining Successful Growth*. Boston: Harvard Business Review Press.

Cooper, R. M., J. A. Pacey, M. J. Bishop, and S. A. McCluskey. 2005. "Early Clinical Experience with a New Videolaryngoscope (GlideScope) in 728 Patients." *Canadian Journal of Anaesthesia* 52: 191–98.

Cochlan, Gregg. 2008. *Love Leadership: What the World Needs Now*. New York: New Voice Press.

Crabtree, Greg. 2014. *Simple Numbers, Straight Talk, Big Profits!: 4 keys to Unlock Your Business Potential*. M J Lane Publishing.

Dobson, Peter. "Theranostics: A Combination of Diagnostics and Therapy." http://www.ema.europa.eu/docs/en_GB/document_library/Presentation/2010/09/WC500096197.pdf

Dr. Seuss. 1990. *Oh, the Places You'll Go!* New York: Random House.

Drucker, Peter F. 2008. *The Essential Drucker: The Best of Sixty Years of Peter Drucker's Essential Writings on Management.* New York: Collins Business Essentials.

Drucker, Peter F. 2008. *Managing Oneself.* Boston: Harvard Business Press.

Fisher, Roger, and William Ury. 2011. *Getting to Yes: Negotiating Agreement without Giving In.* Rev. ed. New York: Penguin Books.

Fishman, Alfred P. 1973. "Shock Lung: A Distinctive Nonentity." *Circulation*, 47 (May): 921–23.

Harnish, Verne. 2002. *Mastering the Rockefeller Habits: What You Must Do to Increase the Value of Your Growing Firm.* Ashburn, Virginia: Gazelles, Inc.

Hsieh, Tony. 2013. *Delivering Happiness: A Path to Profits, Passion, and Purpose.* New York: Grand Central Publishing.

Kim, W. Chan, and Renee Mauborgne. 2005. *Blue Ocean Strategy: How to Create Uncontested Market Space and Make Competition Irrelevant.* Boston: Harvard Business Review Press.

Klock, P. Allan Jr. 2013. "Educating Physician Anesthesiologists to Better Manage Patients with a Difficult Airway." *ASA Newsletter* 77: 18

Mark, Margaret, and Carol Pearson. 2001. *The Hero and the Outlaw: Building Extraordinary Brands through the Power of Archetypes.* New York: McGraw-Hill.

Moore, Geoffrey. 2011. *Crossing the Chasm: Marketing and Selling Disruptive Products to Mainstream Customers.* New York: Harper Business Essentials.

Mullins, John. 2014. *The Customer-Funded Business: Start, Finance, or Grow Your Company with Your Customers' Cash.* New York: Wiley.

Osterwalder, Alexander. Business Model Generation 2010: Wiley

Pacey, John. Allen. 2012. "GlideScope Video Laryngoscope in Military Medicine and Veterans Administration HealthCare." *The Year in Veterans Affairs & Military Medicine.* Tampa, Florida: Faircount Media Group.

Smart, Brad. 2012. *Topgrading.* 3rd ed. New York: Portfolio.

Susko, Shannon Berne. 2014. *The Metronome Effect: The Journey to Predictable Profit.* Charleston, South Carolina: Advantage Media Group.

Taleb, Nassim. 2012. *Antifragile: Things That Gain from Disorder.* New York: Random House.

Thomke, Stefan H. 2003. *Experimentation Matters: Unlocking the Potential of New Technologies for Innovation.* Boston: Harvard Business Review Press.

Yoffie, David, and Michael Cusumano. 2014. *Strategy Rules: Five Timeless Lessons from Bill Gates, Andy Grove, and Steve Jobs.* New York: HarperCollins.

Vaida, Sonia. J., Diana Gaitini, Bruce Ben-David, Mostafa Somri, Carin A. Hagberg, and Luis A. Gaitini. 2004. "A New Supraglottic Airway, the Elisha Airway Device: A Preliminary Study." *Anesthesia & Analgesia,* 99: 124

APPENDIX 1

THE PERFECT MEDICAL PRODUCT CHECKLIST

- The product solves a significant pain point for the customer.
- The product and business model are affordable to the customer and substantially improves patient care, preferably with a large market opportunity.
- The product must work cost effectively for the physician, the hospital or clinic, and the patient and reduce cost.
- The product sale price must have an eightfold margin over the cost of goods to generate the cash required for company growth and the costs of selling.
- The product must enjoy pull from the market to power through the "valley of death" (Geoffrey Moore's "chasm").
- The product originality must allow the company to build a picket fence of patent protection.
- The product must be compliant with FDA, Health Canada, and regulatory bodies.
- The product must obtain a reimbursement code from government or private insurers.
- The product should be rugged and have a long life cycle.
- The product should have online user configurable software updates.

- The product should, ideally, be part of a smart system that learns and configures itself to be antifragile so that it grows custom capacity to make up for user variability.
- The product capital equipment piece anchors the system and creates a bond between customer and company.
- The product single-use components provide a continuous revenue stream for the company and further reinforce the bond between customer and company while providing added convenience and value to the customer. Time produces more revenue as users use devices more as part of the work stream and as more users adopt the product.
- The revenue stream from single-use components lasts well beyond the sale of the last capital equipment devices and may include a subscription business model.
- The product extension paths based on the invention use the same central idea to develop separate, new revenue streams.
- The company must maintain a continuous product-specific quality improvement program even though this is expensive.

APPENDIX 2

Business Model Canvas

Concept tool for start-up company founders with nine key fields to be considered when generating a new business model.

Key Partners	Key Activities	Value Propositions	Customer Relationships	Customer Segments
	Key Resources		Channels	
Cost Structure			Revenue Streams	

Printed in the USA
CPSIA information can be obtained
at www.ICGtesting.com
JSHW012029140824
68134JS00033B/2960

9 781599 326665